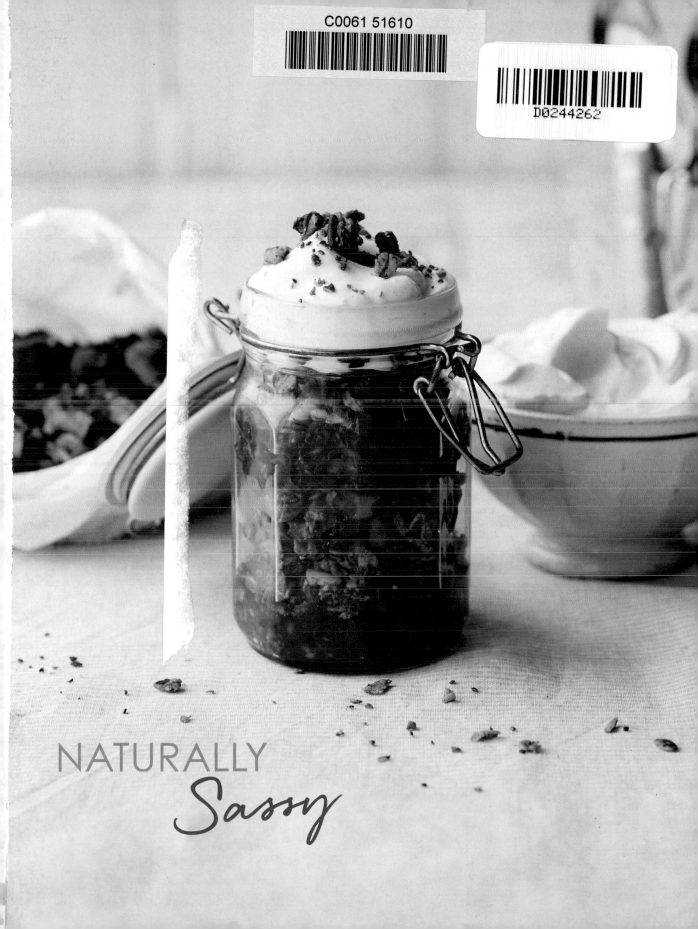

NATURALLY
Sassy

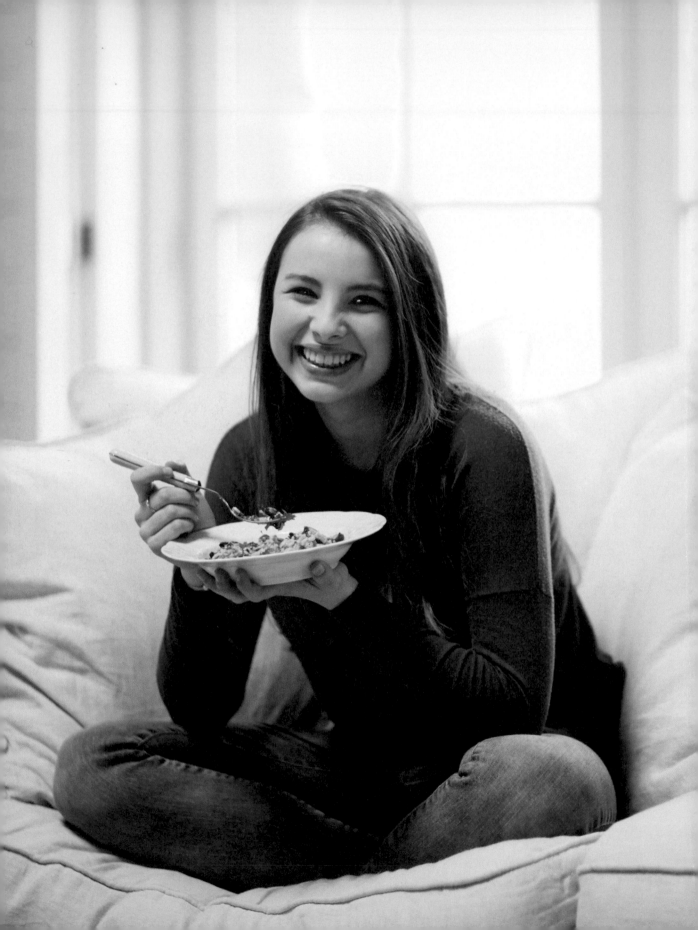

NATURALLY
Sassy

SASKIA GREGSON-WILLIAMS

EBURY
PRESS

10 9 8 7 6 5 4 3 2 1

Ebury Press, an imprint of Ebury Publishing,
20 Vauxhall Bridge Road,
London, SW1V 2SA

Ebury Press is part of the Penguin Random House group
of companies whose addresses can be found at global.
penguinrandomhouse.com

 Penguin
Random House
UK

First published by Ebury Press in 2015

www.eburypublishing.co.uk

A CIP catalogue record for this book is available
from the British Library

Design: Smith & Gilmour
Photography: Matt Russell
Food stylist: Ellie Jarvis
Stylist: Lydia Brun

ISBN: 9781785030970

Colour origination by Altaimage
Printed and bound by L.E.G.O

Penguin Random House is committed to a sustainable
future for our business, our readers and our planet.
This book is made from Forest Stewardship Council®
certified paper.

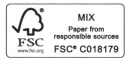

CONTENTS

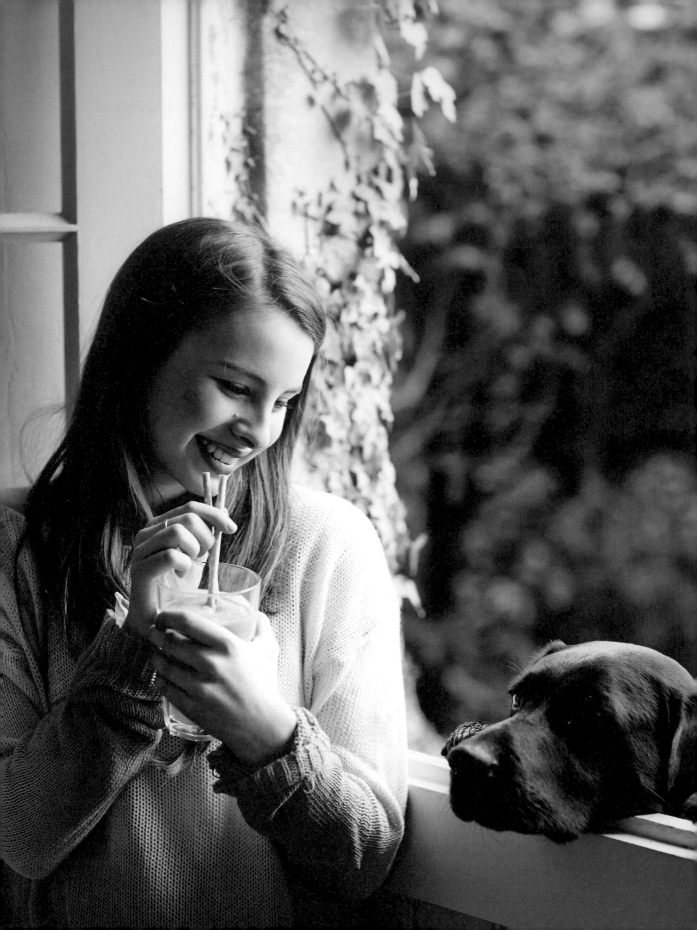

INTRODUCTION

I'm on a mission to show people that the food that does you the most good can be the most delicious and, better still, effortless to prepare. Yes, you heard me right: no more slaving away in the kitchen, running around from shop to shop for 'specialist' health ingredients you've never even heard of, or forking out all your earnings on superfoods! This is the book I so desperately needed not so long ago when the 'how to' of healthy eating was a mystery to me. Sure, I had a few recipe books, but none that told me how I could eat well in a way that would not only be easy and affordable but realistic, something I could do every day of the week. As a ballerina, I have discovered the hard way that food is as important to the body as the training is, and I have had to learn how to make being healthy simple enough to fit into my everyday routine.

How I Learned About Food

The demands of a career as a ballet dancer forced me to grow up quickly. At the age of thirteen, I took my GCSEs so that I could focus exclusively on ballet for the next few crucial years. I moved out of home at a really young age, which brings with it its responsibilities, the biggest being cooking for myself. Like most teenaged girls, I didn't really have any idea about nutrition. I knew my carbs from my protein, but hadn't a clue about what those foods actually did. From my thirteen-year-old perspective, carbs made me fat and protein made me strong.

With image such a vital part of ballet, I found myself counting calories to stay skinny and filling myself with low-fat, low-calorie foods. But my body couldn't take it: I experienced burnout; chronic muscle fatigue; numerous serious injuries, followed by months of rehabilitation; acute inflammation in my joints and muscles, resulting in (far too) many steroid injections; chronic eczema from constant stress; and, to cap it all, campylobacter – a type of food poisoning – which kept me in bed for weeks. At the time, it just seemed like one unfortunate event after the other, but now, in hindsight, it is strikingly clear that my diet was at the root of all of these problems. The type of fuel we use is reflected in the power of the engine, and as you can see, mine had just enough to let me crawl along in first gear!

When I recovered from the food poisoning, after half a year of taking antibiotics, lying in bed watching TV and gorging on chocolate, I came to see that I simply had to do something about what I was eating. I started to understand the relationship between inflammation and illness – that they are closely linked (see 'My Food Philosophy' on page 8 for more on this). So the huge issue I faced during this time was how to get rid of excess inflammation, which I believed to be the root cause and main factor behind all the problems I had encountered that year.

The next revelation was how directly the diet can affect the body and its role in inflammation and subsequent illness. I learned how certain acidic foods encourage inflammation while alkaline foods promote all-round health (for more on this, see pages 8–9). The way forward became clear, and I made it my goal to reclaim my health.

I studied nutrition, read every scientific and nutritional report related to inflammation I could lay my hands on and started having a go in the kitchen, cooking up healthy recipes I found on blogs, in books and magazines. In six months, I went from living in a sugar coma – utterly depressed and keeping myself going on low-calorie, sugar-loaded protein bars and energy drinks – to being high on health, and loving every aspect of my life. I cut out meat, dairy products and anything containing gluten or sugar, and ate more vegetables, fruit, nuts, seeds and gluten-free grains. I found that these swaps completely changed my life, improving my performance as an athlete tenfold.

At first it wasn't that easy – cutting out all these foods at the same time inevitably made me feel lethargic and groggy. Could I eat in this new way and feel my best? It took some fine-tuning to establish a proper balance and make sure I included all the nutrients I needed. But perseverance paid off and all the changes, little and big, came together to transform my outlook on food.

I started experimenting in the kitchen, and discovered a passion for cooking, developing recipes that not only tasted good but targeted the problem I was facing on any particular day, from sore muscles and fatigue to inflamed skin. You name it, I was in the kitchen concocting a remedy! My family and friends were intrigued and began to take an interest, implementing this new approach to food within their own lives and reaping the benefits. It soon became clear that, though this approach was being tested in pretty extreme conditions – as a dancer, I train for eight hours a day – the principles could work for anyone, regardless of their lifestyle.

Following a plant-based diet gives you a feeling of greater clarity and alertness. You'll have more energy and sleep better; your skin will be clearer, you'll lose excess weight and have a better digestion, with no bloating.

Seeing the transformation that this way of eating has made in my life and the lives of people close to me, I wanted to make what I have learned available to everyone, which is why I started my blog Naturally Sassy – and now written a book. I aim to make changing the way you eat easy, attainable and completely undaunting. I want to take food back to basics: simple, healthy, plant-based recipes, full of unprocessed natural ingredients that taste great. While 'delicious' is the bottom line for all my recipes, I hope to show that what we eat has so much more to it than basic refuelling.

My Food Philosophy

I often get asked: 'What's your thing? Is it carb-/gluten-free, vegan?' Healthwise, labelling the way you eat doesn't mean a thing, as while you can be 'everything-free' and appear to lead a very healthy lifestyle, you can actually be filling yourself with rubbish. My philosophy is to eat only unrefined, plant-based, natural food that does your body nothing but good. Purposeful eating is something I base all my recipes and meals around, using ingredients that heal, strengthen, reduce inflammation and increase energy – or target any other problems I may be facing on a particular day.

Acidic Foods and Inflammation

For most of us, the sad fact is that what we eat doesn't give us the best chance of feeling the best we can. The processed foods that make up the majority of the western diet leave us feeling lethargic, groggy, bloated and constantly on the edge of getting ill. Meat, dairy products and foods containing gluten or sugar are all 'acidic foods' – that is, they have an acidic effect on the body when they are digested, triggering inflammation, the body's response to harmful stimuli. This makes us more prone to disease, for inflammation is at the root of nearly every physical ailment. Acne, flu, headaches, cramp, bloating, cardiovascular disease, cancer, you name it – inflammation is the cause or a big contributing factor. Why would I choose to eat food that made me feel groggy or weakened my immune system? When a close family member contracted breast cancer and, in recovery, was told to completely cut out acidic dairy products and red meat, as well as limiting any meat or fish intake, it really hit home. Why wait for something to happen when you could prevent it, by simply eating well? This example is taken from the extreme end of the spectrum, but if simply by eating natural food you gain a better perspective and outlook on life as well as a stronger immune system and more energy – then why wouldn't you go for it?

Power of Plants

'Alkaline foods', by contrast, do the opposite – they have 'alkalising' effect when they are digested, creating a balanced environment in the body. These include vegetables, fruits, nuts, seeds and gluten-free grains – all ingredients that I use in this book. Unrefined, plant-based foods are easier for the body to digest and hence provide the best source of energy, enabling us to feel focused and alert and banishing those energy rollercoasters that refined foods take us on. As well as being delicious, they contain vital vitamins and minerals that can help the body in many different ways. Each has a number of key nutrients that act as natural remedies to help nourish, strengthen and protect you. It's important that, when you're planning a meal, you take into account what your body really needs. With this in mind, I've included a section at the back of the book, 'Foods for Health', to help guide you through the properties of various plant-based foods I've used in the recipes here. That way, you can be your own pharmacist, and prescribe yourself the recipe that is best suited to you. You may also like to look through my pantry essentials on page 14 for a list of basic store-cupboard items that I use every day.

Foods to Eliminate

While I always prefer to think about the foods I'll be adding to my diet, eating naturally does mean we have to get rid of a few too. Meat, dairy products and foods containing gluten or refined sugar all generally make us feel less than our best and should be phased out. While it may sound pretty daunting to have to reduce and eventually cut out all these foods, over time you'll find that it is nowhere near as limiting as it might appear at first. But before you start to implement any changes, it's really important you know why you are doing this.

Meat

One of the chief reasons we think eating lots of meat is beneficial to our bodies is because of its abundance of protein. Protein is needed to build, repair and aid muscle growth. It's known to be the main food group dieters focus on because it is broken down and digested slowly, which gives you the feeling of being fuller for longer, staving off hunger pangs. The downside is that meat requires a lot of hard work by your body to break down into energy. Plant-based protein is broken down far more easily, and there are many rich sources, including brown rice, quinoa, nuts, seeds, pulses and legumes. Eating these will leave you feeling much less lethargic, as the body, instead of having to expend energy on lengthy digestion, is able to function far more efficiently. You will still be supplying your body with all the protein it needs and it will benefit you far, far more. If you must eat meat, have it as a treat, not a staple, and buy the best quality. This ideally means free range, organic and locally sourced.

Dairy

I grew up with chronic eczema all over my body, and only when I cut out dairy foods did it disappear, showing the huge intolerance I had to them. This is in fact one of the most common food groups to cause intolerances. Much non-organic dairy produce is also loaded with hormones and antibiotics that were given to the cow, or simply added to the milk to preserve it – additives that are absorbed into your bloodstream with adverse effects on your health, from acne and bloating to eczema and stomach cramps. If you love the taste of milk and cheese, there are fortunately lots of dairy-free alternatives. I substitute cow's milk with almond, oat or rice milk, cream and ice cream with delicious blends of cashews and coconut milk or oil, and cheese with a creamy fusion of nuts and nutritional yeast.

Gluten

A mixture of two proteins, gluten is present in cereal grains, especially wheat. Gluten is a common cause of abdominal pain, bloating, gas, anaemia, depression, joint pain and muscle cramps. Because of the wide range of symptoms, it is easy to be gluten-intolerant without realising it, and blame the symptoms on another cause. For me, a gluten-free diet has completely changed the way my body feels, relieving muscle tightness and boosting energy levels. Grains containing gluten include wheat-based pastas, flours and breads, breakfast cereals, couscous, bulgur wheat and (if to a lesser degree) rolled oats. But there are tons of delicious alternatives that are gluten-free, from grains like quinoa, buckwheat, brown rice and millet to flours made from rice, coconut and buckwheat. Gluten-free rolled oats are available too. Much easier to digest, these foodstuffs are all far healthier than their gluten-full counterparts!

Refined Sugar

I could rant all day about sugar, and while the media are only just cottoning on to the negative effects of this legal drug, its addictive properties continue to lure us, with sugary products saturating our supermarkets. Unlike other 'drugs', no one speaks about overdosing on sugar, but these grains of sweetness cause a host of health problems from weight gain and skin conditions to high cholesterol. In the long term, this sweet poison weakens your immune system, paving the way for serious disease. It's no secret that I have a huge sweet tooth and to keep it happy I use unrefined sweeteners such as agave and pure maple syrup, Medjool dates or raw honey. These are unrefined sugars with a lower GI that deliver a more steady flow of energy. They're not supplying empty calories but fibre, vitamins and minerals that are beneficial to the body. In my sweet recipes, I try to offset these sweeteners with sufficient protein and fibre from other ingredients to balance sugar levels in the body to stave off a post-indulgence sugar crash.

Using This Book

The aim of this book, and the recipes in it, is to encourage you to eat purposefully, preparing food that is the best for you. I want to show you how to make a breakfast that starts you off properly; easy lunches you can eat in or pack for work; speedy weekday dinners or meals to linger over with friends and family; energising snacks to eat before a workout or to carry with you for a healthy boost. Your body needs different fuel to do different things: whether that's to increase your stamina, fight injury or infection. If you have a job interview, a big date or any other occasion you want to look fantastic for, you should eat the right things for that too. Every recipe you make should have a nutritional benefit for your body and be tailored to what you need for that day.

Although designed so that anybody can start to make the tiny steps they need to make their diet healthier, this book aims to completely change the way you view what's on your plate, and the relationship you have with your food. It's not about counting calories or denying yourself the pleasure of eating delicious dishes; it's about being fit rather than thin for the sake of it, strong rather than skinny, and happy rather than guilty. This way of eating gives you the best platform for a toned athletic body. But it will also make everyone who tries it look and feel better, even if they only dip their toe in.

The book contains around 120 plant-based recipes that are designed to support you through every step of the day. Whether you're at home or on the go, relaxed or in a rush, I hope to make this way of eating affordable and effortless. The recipe chapters are interspersed with 'How To' sections to show you the basic principles for making some of the recipes, from porridge to a 'balance' bowl (see pages 38–39 and 158–159), so that, in time, you'll be able to make them without thinking and using a whole range of different ingredients. With these sections, I want you to put on your chef hat and get experimenting!

You'll also find each chapter has an array of recipes suited to different days. In 'Breakfast' you'll find recipes you can make in 5 minutes the night before and grab before you leave in the morning, dishes that will take no more than 15 minutes to prepare but leave you feeling ready for the day ahead, and weekend brunch recipes – healthy twists on the classic more indulgent type of breakfast.

In 'Soups and Salads' you'll not only find quick and easy lunch recipes, but a guide on how to make healthy lunches 'to go'. This section shows you the foods you can prep up to a week ahead, and how simple it can be to compile a health-tastic lunch every day.

In 'Mains' I've really tried to make every recipe as affordable and simple to make as possible, dividing them into sections – 'One-Pot Wonders', '15-minute Meals', '45-minute or Less' and 'Dressed to Impress' – to give a realistic idea of how quick they are to prepare, and what sort of occasion they are best suited to. For those times when you need a little extra something to see you through the day, there is 'Savoury Snacks and Sweet Treats', while 'Desserts' contains a whole range of healthy yet delicious puddings.

Throughout the book, I've included notes and tips to help you prepare a particular recipe. I've also made sure, where possible, to mention a few simple ingredient swaps you might like to make, to give you a bit of artistic licence to pick and choose your favourites/whatever you may have in the fridge.

How to Get Started in 5, 4, 3, 2, 1!

When you're so used to eating certain foods, but want to wean yourself off them, it's not only your tastebuds you have to contend with, but your routine – the hardest thing to break. When I overhauled my diet, I cut out everything overnight. It was a big challenge as I battled with massive cravings, headaches, lethargy and grogginess. My body went into serious detox mode – testament to all the rubbish I had been eating! While I have always been very impatient and want everything to happen yesterday, this really isn't the best way to make a lifelong change. Little steps each day are key, and before you know it, those small changes will result in that one big transformation you've been wanting – stress- and craving-free! If I could tell the Sassy I was four years ago what I know now – I would tell her that the best way to get started is in five steps. While I can't go back and save myself those struggles, hopefully I can spare you:

1. Pimp Your Kitchen
The hardest thing when you're removing processed foods from your diet is to have them still lurking around your kitchen. The first step to eating well is to prepare to eat well.

~ Kit your fridge out with healthy ingredients: fresh vegetables, dairy-free milks, coconut yoghurt, fresh berries – the list of what you can munch on is endless. Get rid of all the sugary snacks and refined carbs so there is nothing left to tempt you.

~ I love buying lots of jars (or recycling old ones) and using them to hold all my nuts, seeds, oats and grains. Visually it's so much more exciting, and also means you can always see how much food you have in the cupboard – so you don't over-buy and, equally, so you'll know when you need more.

~ The final thing you can do is invest in a few kitchen tools and pieces of equipment to make your healthy eating that much more delicious. My top three have to be my spiraliser, food processor and blender. You don't need these but they make life so much easier. A good food processor and high-powered blender can be a little expensive, but there are some reasonably priced brands that work wonders too (see my website, www.naturallysassy.co.uk, for more details). A juicer is lovely to have, but not essential, while a nut-milk bag comes in very handy if you're making your own dairy-free milk (see pages 74–75). If you don't want to invest in a spiraliser just yet, a vegetable peeler makes a good substitute. You won't get the same spaghetti strands but you can create wide pappardelle ribbons. There are now quite a few different spiralisers on the market and some are pretty affordable. Once you start spiralising, you will use this tool constantly, I can assure you! It makes vegetables into spaghetti – see my Courgette noodles with a sun-dried pasta sauce on page 125 for an example!

2. Simple Swaps
It all starts with a few simple swaps that can take your diet from C class to A in a matter of bites! While some of these may be obvious, they're all so important.

GRAINS
White/wholemeal bread >>> Gluten-free buckwheat or quinoa bread
White rice >>> Brown rice
Couscous >>> Quinoa
Wholewheat pasta >>> Brown rice pasta
Egg noodles >>> Buckwheat noodles
Breakfast cereals >>> Gluten-free muesli/oats, brown rice puffs

DAIRY
Cow's milk >>> Brown rice, almond, oat or coconut milk
Cream >>> Coconut cream
Butter >>> Coconut/olive oil, dairy-free coconut butter

SWEETENERS
Sugar >>> Raw honey, agave or pure maple syrup
Chocolate >>> Raw chocolate

3. Get Creative
There's nothing worse than a bland plate of food – not only does it put you in a pretty grumpy mood, it certainly doesn't get you excited about healthy eating! I would say being creative with what you eat is one of the most important things you can do. When I first started eating a plant-based diet, I ate the same meals every single day – and it was tiresome. This book is bursting with delicious recipes for you to try, allowing you to ring the changes each and every day – a brilliant starting point for getting creative in the kitchen. Use my 'How To' sections to customise your own dishes too.

And share your thoughts and creations online, whether that means starting a blog or social media page. Sharing your experiences won't just help you stick to your new food regime, but will also help inspire others to do the same. It's wonderful to connect to like-minded foodies or those who are experiencing similar challenges to you. I'd love to see what you've made from this book, so Tweet or Instagram me @naturallysassy_.

4. Prepare
Preparation is key. While time may be of the essence, that shouldn't mean unhealthy ready meals. Putting aside just a bit of time on a Sunday, you can make eating when you're out and about effortless. I always spend an hour each Sunday morning to prep an array of salads for picking and mixing during the week (see pages 109–111). I pile a spoonful of each salad into my lunch box to enjoy between ballet sessions and meetings. I also like to whizz up some gingerbread or brownie bars (see page 172) to snack on during the week. If I'm feeling on top of things, I'll also get a head start with breakfast and do a batch of Overnight oats (see pages 46–47), so I can assemble a serving with some fresh berries the night before. Believe it or not, this doesn't take much time at all, especially when you get in the swing of things!

5. Get Friends and Family Involved

Food can be used for comfort, to build muscle, lose fat or simply fuel the body, but the real definition of a good meal is one enjoyed with the people you love. When embarking on a lifestyle change, it's great not only to have the support of those around you, but also get them involved too. Pick a few recipes from the book and plan when you're going to make them – have fun playing around with the recipes and then sit down and enjoy what you've made together. When you're having a good time, your body relaxes and you digest food more easily, maximising the amount of nutrition you get from the food. Preparing a meal to enjoy with friends and family also means you'll tend to select the food with greater care and eat at a steadier pace in their company, helping digestion and nutrient absorption.

My Pantry

To eat well, you have to have good food to hand, which is why I always try and keep my kitchen stocked up with a variety of healthy ingredients. I've put together a list of kitchen essentials for you to keep in mind when you're planning your weekly shop (opposite). While I don't buy all of them at once, I try to make sure I have a wide range of the basic foods (pulses, grains, beans, brown rice pasta, buckwheat noodles, tinned tomatoes, coconut cream) that have a long shelf life, so I always have these to hand, then the rest I tend to buy once I've planned what I'll be making that week. I find planning what you're going to be eating/making is so much more cost-effective – that way you never over-buy. It's also a big help when it comes to making good food choices, as you're not reduced to making a hasty decision when you're starving!

I hope this guide will help give you a basic idea of the foods to stock up on in addition to fresh fruit and vegetables. Eat and enjoy these foods and your body will thank you for it. For any products you haven't heard of, or want to know where I buy them from, see my website.

Secrets of the Superfoods

I love hosting Naturally Sassy dinner parties. It's really fun to see how amazed people are to discover that the delicious meal they're eating is so good for them. I get tons of questions about the ingredients in each dish and everyone's always so intrigued when they hear about foods like cacao powder (they assume I'm just mispronouncing cocoa!). Because these 'superfoods' may not be familiar to you, I thought I'd better explain a little more about them.

A superfood is a foodstuff that, gram for gram, contains more nutrients than other foods, with greater benefits to health. Many are made into a powder, which not only helps you gauge the serving size but makes it very easy to add them to drinks, including smoothies and juices, and different dishes. The only downside is that they can be pricey, but, on the other hand, they do last for ages.

If you can't afford to spend money on these foods, don't worry – they are by no means essential in any of my recipes. If you can, I suggest buying two or three of those below, see how you like them and, most of all, how they make you feel. My top three to get you going would be cacao powder, chia seeds and spirulina.

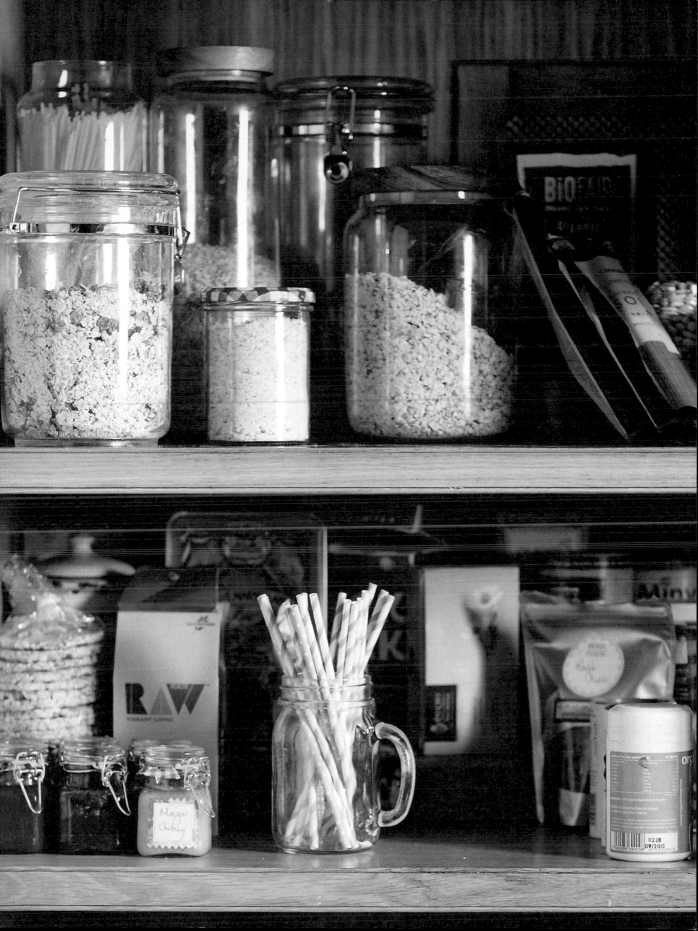

KITCHEN ESSENTIALS

Dairy-free milks

Oat milk
Almond milk
Brown rice milk
Coconut milk,
    coconut cream and
    coconut water

Nut and seed butters

Almond butter
Cashew butter
Peanut butter
Hazelnut butter
Pumpkin seed butter
Tahini (sesame seed butter)

Nut and seeds

Almonds
Cashews
Hazelnuts
Pecans
Brazil nuts
Walnuts
Pistachios
Pine nuts
Desiccated/shredded
    coconut
Pumpkin seeds
Sesame seeds
Sunflower seeds
Hemp seeds
Chia Seeds
Poppy seeds
Flaxseeds

Grains

Quinoa
Millet
Buckwheat
Brown rice
Amaranth
Wild rice
Oats (can be gluten-free)
Millet flakes
Pasta, noodles and bread
Brown rice pasta
Buckwheat noodles
Mung bean fettucine
Buckwheat bread

Flours and baking ingredients

Brown rice
Buckwheat
Ground almonds
Coconut flour
Chickpea flour
    (gram or besan flour)
Cacao (or cocoa) powder
Cacao nibs
Baking powder
Bicarbonate of soda

Natural sweeteners

Agave syrup
Pure maple syrup
Raw/manuka honey

Pulses (dried and tinned)

Lentils (beluga,
    split red, Puy)
Kidney beans
Black beans
Chickpeas

Tinned/bottled fruit and vegetables

Tomatoes (whole
    and chopped)
Passata
Olives
Apple purée

Dried fruit

Sultanas
Raisins
Apricots
Goji berries
Medjool dates

Oils and condiments

Olive oil (extra-virgin
    for dressings)
Coconut oil
Apple cider vinegar
Tamari sauce
Miso paste
Natural salt (such
    as pink Himalayan)
Black peppercorns
    and other spices
Dried herbs
Vegetable stock cubes
    and bouillon powder

Acai Berry

Acai berry, from a tropical plant in the Amazon, comes in powdered and capsule form and is an incredible source of antioxidants, boosting your immune system and protecting your body against damaging free radicals. It is also rich in essential fatty acids omega-3 and -6 and contains omega-9 oleic acid, making it a true beauty food.
How to use: Add this to smoothies and breakfast bowls (see pages 35, 78 and 82).

Baobab Powder

Baobab powder is wonderfully sweet and tastes a little like sherbet. It contains an abundance of vitamin C and malic acid, which have strong energy-enhancing properties. It also helps you absorb and convert food to energy more efficiently.
How to use: Adding some to your smoothies will give you an awesome sweet energy boost! I also love stirring it into creamy bowls of porridge, or using it to enhance the 'super' status of my raw energy bars.

Bee Pollen

Bee pollen, made by honey bees, is considered to be one of nature's most nourishing and complete foods as it contains almost all the nutrients required by our bodies. It's richer in protein than any other animal source, contains more amino acids than the likes of eggs, beef or cheese, and is rich in vitamin B and folic acid. Bee pollen and raw/manuka honey are the two foods that I do eat outside of a vegan diet.
How to use: Add to smoothies and hot chocolate (see pages 78–82 and 76) or sprinkle on porridge and smoothie bowls (see pages 38–45 and 28–35).

Cacao Nibs

While cacao nibs look like chocolate chips, don't be fooled. They have a distinctive personality of their own and are very, very bitter – an acquired taste that becomes incredibly addictive! Cacao nibs are derived from cacao, the completely unprocessed form of chocolate. This means that, like cacao powder, they still contain all the wonderful minerals and vitamins that are normally lost in the cooking process.
How to use: Because of their bitterness, I love to use cacao nibs to garnish something very sweet, such as my smoothie bowls (see pages 28–35). Just a few sprinkled on top is delicious.

Cacao Powder

Made by cold-pressing unroasted cocoa beans, raw cacao is the pure, unprocessed form of chocolate that comes just as nature intended it, with all its vitamins and minerals intact. Cacao is one of the world's best sources of antioxidants, helping fight inflammation in the body and making it an incredible immune booster. It also helps to raise your levels of serotonin, meaning that it can act as a natural mood enhancer and antidepressant.
How to use: Cacao powder is amazing in any chocolatey dessert. I also add it to my porridge and always end the day with a Superfood Hot Chocolate (see page 76)! In my recipes, you can substitute with standard cocoa powder, bearing in mind that it is not a superfood as many of the nutrients will have been lost during processing.

Chia Seeds

Chia seeds are a great source of protein for

vegetarians, with the added benefit that they don't have any cholesterol. A 28g serving of these little super seeds contains around 4.5g of protein, which is nearly 10 per cent of the daily recommended intake. They're also the highest plant source of omega-3 fatty acids, vital for maintaining a healthily functioning heart. They also help to lower blood pressure and cholesterol, reducing your risk of heart disease and strokes.

How to use: You can add these to smoothie bowls or Overnight oats (see pages 28–35 and 46–51) or, my favourite, use them as an egg replacement in baking, as I do for my brownies (see page 192). For one 'egg', you simply mix 1 tablespoon of chia seeds with 3 tablespoons of water and let the mixture sit for 15 minutes before incorporating it into the rest of the cake batter.

Chlorella Powder

A type of green algae, chlorella is brimming with liver-detoxing and -cleansing properties. It helps to promote good digestion, clear skin, strong hair and nails. It's also full of blood-boosting iron and high in vitamins B6 and B12.
How to use: Add to a green smoothie or green juice (see pages 30–32 and 80).

Goji Berries

Goji berries are another superfood that can take a few bites to get used to, I, for one, love the sweet and tangy taste. One cool fact about goji berries is that they contain 18 amino acids, making them the fruit with the highest protein concentration. They have a whopping ten times more antioxidant capacity than blueberries, and have also been shown to have 15 times the amount of iron found in spinach.

How to use: Add to muesli (see page 65) and salads, or sprinkle on top of porridge and smoothie bowls (see pages 38–39 and 28–31).

Lucuma Powder

Made from a Peruvian fruit traditionally known as the 'Gold of the Incas', lucuma powder has huge nutritional benefits. It is high in carotene, a powerful antioxidant that rejuvenates the body and reduces the effects of ageing. It's also rich in iron and fibre, essential for good digestion.
How to use: Add to desserts and smoothies as a natural sweetener. It would make a perfect addition to my 'caramel' protein smoothie (see page 79).

Maca Powder

Grown in Peru, maca is a root belonging to the radish family long prized for its health benefits. It is high in phosphorus and manganese, as well as iron – promoting healthy circulation and increasing energy levels, thereby helping to boost strength and stamina.
How to use: Maca powder has a very strong taste, which is never very nice on its own and therefore best disguised by adding to dishes with a good, strong flavour of their own. I love to add it to my Chocolate overnight oats and warming Chocolate porridge (see pages 48 and 44).

Nutritional Yeast

Despite it's somewhat unappetising name, nutritional yeast is the perfect answer to any cheese cravings when you're eating a vegan diet. These flakes are not only bursting with flavour, but nutrients too. They are full of B vitamins, making nutritional yeast an invaluable source of plant-based protein (see pages 10 and 20–21). Ensuring you have enough protein is so important when you're not eating meat – just adding a sprinkling of these flakes to various dishes is a great way to up your intake.

How to use: Make into nut cheeses, add to risottos (see page 149) or sprinkle over gluten-free pasta and other hot dishes.

Spirulina Powder

I'm not going to lie – spirulina powder is pretty disgusting on its own. It tastes a little like I imagine pond weed would – hardly surprising as it is in fact an algae. Spirulina contains a wealth of beta-carotene, chlorophyll, iron and vitamin B6, which help to support and strengthen your immune system. The powder also contains around 70 per cent of its weight in protein, including all the essential amino acids. This means it is a fantastic addition to a plant-based diet, especially before and after a workout.

How to use: To hide the slightly unpleasant taste, I always add it to a sweet green smoothie. While the colour of the drink may become darker, it won't affect the taste.

Wheatgrass Powder

You've probably heard of wheatgrass in its more pungent form – a wheatgrass shot. Wheatgrass contains an amazing amount of chlorophyll, which helps cleanse the body of harmful toxins. High in fibre, it is also beneficial for the digestive system. No wonder that a few years ago gym-goers and healthistas were downing them like there was no tomorrow. Now wheatgrass is being sold in powdered form, it's much easier to enjoy.

How to use: Wheatgrass is high in energy-metabolising enzymes and minerals, so add it to your green smoothie first thing for a boost of energy!

Get to Know the Food Groups

Food groups can be one of the most confusing topics in nutrition to discuss, as everyone has a very different opinion. Initially, I found navigating my way around the whole issue, deciding which were the 'right' and 'wrong' foods, pretty difficult, and without meat in the picture, I had no idea how I was going to get my proper quota of protein.

Equally, with a greasy burger or a bag of fries strictly off limits, I was confused about what sort of fat to eat, and even more confused as to why I needed it. When I began to study nutrition, it was a real eye opener, showing the components of what makes up our diet in a very different light. Before changing my diet, I was eating very high-protein diet meals with lots of vegetables but minimal carbohydrates and fats. From what I'd previously learned, I believed that carbohydrates and fat make you fat. Those food groups seemed like the enemy and something I instinctively ran away from. And, talking to other people, I realised I wasn't alone in this: it seems we're brought up thinking that we need to cut certain food groups out in order to look and feel our best. This simply isn't the case.

Food groups are designed to work in synergy: without one, you will lack the essential vitamins and minerals your body needs. Of course there are the high-GI 'bad' carbs and saturated fats (see below) that we can all live without, but unrefined, complex carbohydrates are an important element in a healthy diet. With diet books left, right and centre sporting the latest fashionable way of fasting, it's easy to get sucked into thinking each food belongs to one category, but in fact most foods consist of an array of nutrients belonging to several food groups. What's more, no two fats, carbs or proteins are the same. Everything I've learned has given me a greater understanding of how the body works, and in particular what suits me as an individual – the foods it feels best on and, most importantly, how to assemble a really well-balanced meal. Below I've gone through the four main food groups to hopefully convey a better idea of what they each do, and why we need each of them.

Carbohydrates

Carbs are the first food we tend to cut out when we're trying to lose weight, and the food group that arouses the most controversy. It's very common to believe all carbs are equal, but that's far from the truth. Carbohydrates come in refined and unrefined forms, which affect how the body uses and absorbs them. Refined carbohydrates – from white bread and rice and pasta to chocolate bars, cakes and soft drinks – as well as having most of their nutrients removed during processing, contain artificial sugars that are broken down very quickly by the body, giving you an instant buzz before an almighty sugar crash. They are highly inflammatory and, over time, can be a key factor in many health problems.

On the other side, we have unrefined, complex carbohydrates – whole grains such as quinoa, buckwheat, oats and millet, as well as dense root vegetables such as potatoes, sweet potatoes and carrots. These are digested and absorbed by the body much more slowly, so that instead of that instant sugar hit, energy is released at a steady pace. Your blood-sugar levels remain on an even keel and you are able to feel the full benefit of the food.

Unrefined carbohydrates should make up 50 per cent of the average diet, and should never be restricted. These carbohydrates are our main source of sustained energy and, without them, we feel weak and lethargic. As an athlete or gym-goer, this is particularly important post-workout to restore your glycogen levels. If you're on a diet, cleanse or weight-loss programme, it is still important to eat moderate amounts of unrefined carbs.

Healthy carbohydrates
Nuts, seeds
Beans, chickpeas, lentils
Brown rice, quinoa, millet, buckwheat
Rolled oats, quinoa flakes, millet flakes
Brown rice spaghetti, rice pasta,
   buckwheat noodles

Protein

Proteins are large molecules consisting of 21 amino acids, essential for healthy bodily function. With a vegan diet, protein is something I get asked about constantly. This is heightened by the fact that I'm a ballet dancer, a very physical career that requires a certain level of protein consumption in order for your muscles to recover after every performance. When I first stopped eating meat, I had no idea about how to substitute it with plant-based protein and instead ate a diet stuffed with refined carbohydrates. Without enough protein in my diet, my muscles felt less flexible and recovered more slowly and I frequently found myself feeling hungry very soon after a big meal. Knowing I needed to include more protein, I started looking into the best ways to do this. It was at this point I discovered how many plant-based foods did contain a good amount of protein, and found that pairing certain foods really helped. Not all foods contain all of the essential 21 amino acids, which is why often combining two high-protein foods can work so well, especially if you consume a variety of these. Below are a list of all the vegetables, pulses and grains that should be on your protein radar.

Amount of protein per serving
Peas – 100g = 5g protein
Kale – 100g = 4.3g protein
Spinach – 100g = 2.9g protein
Broccoli – 100g = 2.8g protein

Lentils – 100g = 9g protein
Chickpeas – 100g = 9g protein
Kidney beans – 100g = 8.5g protein
Split peas – 100g = 8g protein
Black beans – 100g = 8g protein

Peanut butter – 2 tablespoons = 8g protein
Tahini – 2 tablespoons = 8g protein
Almond butter – 2 tablespoons = 6g protein
Cashew butter – 2 tablespoons = 6g protein

Almonds – 25g = 5.2g protein
Sunflower seeds – 25g = 5.2g protein
Pumpkin seeds – 25g = 4.8g protein
Cashews – 25g = 4.5g protein
Brazil nuts – 25g = 3.5g protein
Pecans – 25g = 2.2g protein

Quinoa – 170g = 7.5g protein
Oats – 40g = 6.8g protein
Brown rice – 170g = 4.4g protein

Nutritional yeast – 10g = 8g protein
Bee pollen – 10g = 2.5g protein
Chia seeds – 10g = 1.7g protein

Fats
Like carbohydrates, fats don't have the best reputation. The words 'low fat' abound on supermarket shelves, giving us all the impression that low fat is better for us. As I've mentioned, food groups work in synergy, creating a healthy environment in the body if you eat a balanced diet. However, as with all food groups, fats aren't all the same. There are saturated fats, like those contained in cheese and butter, and unsaturated fats such as those found in avocados, nuts, seeds and olive oil. With the exception of coconut oil, saturated fats are very acidic and hard to digest, and over time they can lead to obesity and inflammation-based illnesses. The same holds true for 'trans' fats – artificially created unsaturated fats found in many commercially prepared foods. Natural unsaturated fats, however, are key to a healthy diet and a toned body. While the word 'fat' doesn't exactly go hand in hand with toning and slimming, it's thought that certain unsaturated fats could actually help to boost your metabolism! These healthy fats have many other benefits: they are full of skin-loving omegas, promoting a glowing skin and a glossy head of hair. Whenever I feel my appearance is less than my best, my remedy is always an avocado!

Fats to Love!
Olive oil, olives
Avocado
Coconut oil, coconut milk/
    cream, coconut flakes
Nuts, seeds and nut and seed butters

How to Source Ingredients

I'm all about delicious organic, locally sourced, seasonal food – of course, who wouldn't be? At the same time I appreciate that, on a day-to-day basis, this isn't realistic. Here I've given a few tips about how best to source ingredients for the recipes in my book, keeping expenses down and the quality up!

When to Buy Organic

Since I can remember, my mum has been preaching about organic food, and always making it her mission to buy totally organic wherever possible. Needless to say, for the best part of my life I ate a totally organic diet – I'm pretty sure my bed sheets were even organic! When I moved away from home and started cooking for myself, I was astounded by how much one meal would cost if I made it with entirely organic ingredients. My shopping bill would be astronomical, even if just for one person.

Thankfully, as more and more people have turned to buying organic produce, the volumes in shops have become much larger and hence costs have gone down. Even so, not everyone can afford to buy organic every day. Personally, while I do always buy certain organic foods, this is never my priority, and nor do I believe it should be yours.

The most important aspect to consider when buying food is the purity. It needs to be pure and unrefined, with no additives or preservatives. You may have heard of the 'dirty dozen' – a list of the most important foods to purchase in organic form due to their pesticide contamination. If you're able to buy anything organic, these should be the ones.

The Dirty Dozen

Apples	Blueberries
Celery	Cucumbers
Grapes	Lettuce
Nectarines	Peaches
Potatoes	Strawberries
Spinach	Sweet peppers

Shopping Seasonally

I often hear chefs and bloggers rave about seasonal produce because of its depth of flavour but, for me, this isn't of prime importance – shopping seasonally is more about being savvy. Buying seasonal food is a great way to keep your shopping costs down, as when different foods are in season, markets, greengrocers and supermarkets have an abundance and the price is greatly reduced. So if you're in the know, this is an easy way to cut down your costs each month. I've listed below the foods you should look out for during the year so you have a great starting point for using seasonal produce in a healthy and delicious way!

Spring (March–May)

Asparagus	Beetroot
Cucumbers	Garlic
Leeks	Little Gem lettuce
Mint	Parsley
Peas	Rocket
Spinach	Strawberries

Summer (June–August)

Asparagus	Carrots
Cauliflower	Celery
Courgettes	Cucumbers
Parsley	Peas
Red cabbage	Romaine lettuce
Spinach	Blueberries
Raspberries	Strawberries

Autumn (September–November)

Carrots	Cauliflower
Celery	Courgettes
Cucumbers	Leeks
Kale	Peas
Potatoes	Red cabbage
Spinach	Apples
Blueberries	Pears

Winter (December–February)

Broccoli	Carrots
Cauliflower	Leeks
Kale	Potatoes

Shopping Online

Online shopping has changed my life. I used to find myself in the supermarket at around 9 p.m., feeling sorry for myself, exhausted and exceedingly hungry – a terrible combination when you're food shopping. This would lead me to buy unhealthy ready meals, simply so that I could fuel myself within the next half an hour! The next morning I would regret my unhealthy choices and the blues would set in, the cycle only to repeat itself the following day. To get myself out of this rut, I tried online shopping, and since then I've never looked back. Online shopping is a great way to stock up on everything you need for the week without even walking out your front door. It means making much better choices, and being able to really plan your recipes and meals, instead of grabbing something on the fly. It proved a saving grace for me, too, when I first tried it, as I found processed food a lot less tempting on a computer screen than in the flesh!

Nowadays, I find online shopping brilliant for time efficiency. I don't have to go out to buy it and instead my shopping is delivered every Sunday morning, meaning that I'm stocked up for the rest of week. It's also a good way of monitoring how much you're spending. Unlike the supermarket, you can see how much everything costs in your shopping basket and add or subtract ingredients as you go. It's also wonderful to be able to see all the special deals on offer at a glance, without actually having to march around a supermarket to find them. There are lots of great online health-food shops, too, ideal if you're looking for a more specialised ingredient that you can't find on the supermarket sites. Being able to buy your groceries like this is a big step forward – a modern way to shop that makes a huge difference! I've listed my favourite online supermarkets on my website. You'll also find details about where to source superfoods and other more unusual ingredients. A few quick clicks and you'll be sorted – well on the way to a healthier you!

Cup Measures

Growing up in the USA, where I first tried my hand at cooking, I was taught to use cup measurements for everything, and I find it far easier than using a set of scales. In this book, I have given you the option of either weighing ingredients or, wherever possible, using cups. Cups are based on US measures (1 cup = 240ml). Rather than using a measuring cup or jug, you could use a small mug instead – maybe measure water into it first to work out its capacity – and providing you use the same mug for measuring every ingredient throughout a recipe, the proportions will be the same and the recipe should work perfectly.

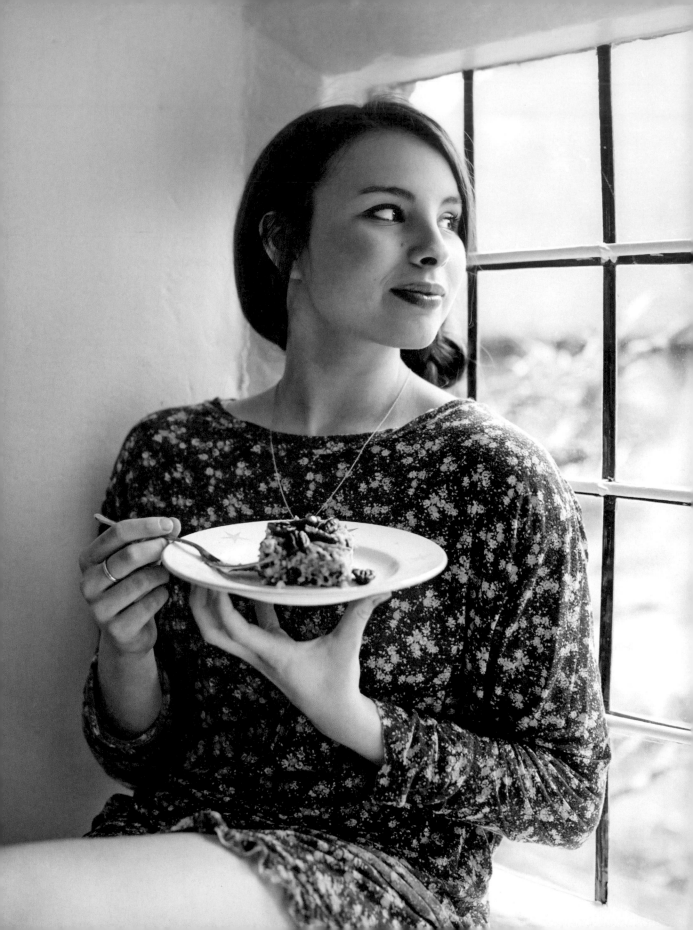

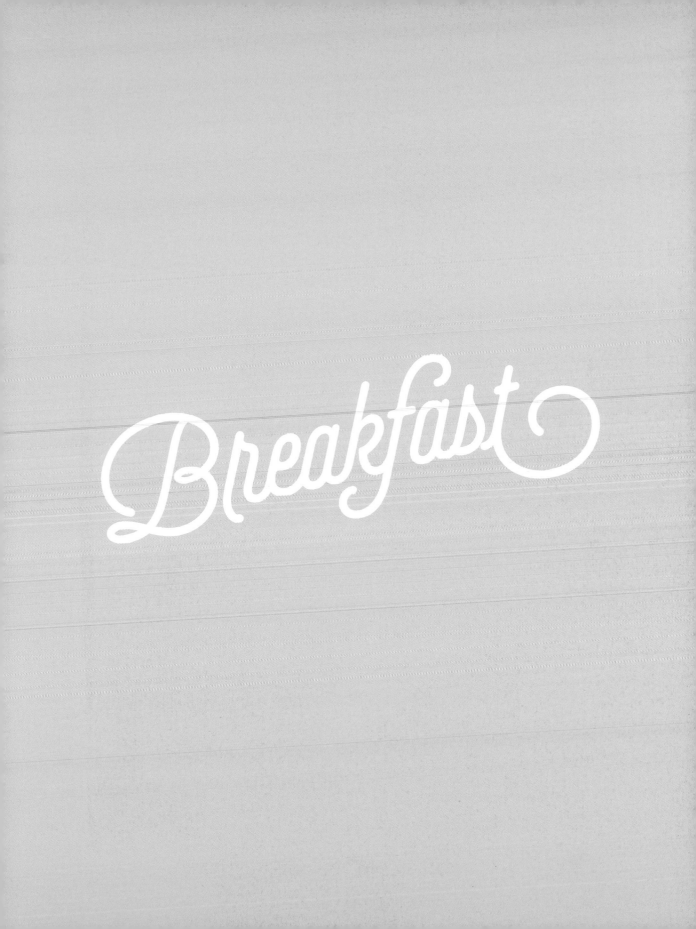

Breakfast is my favourite meal of the day and, as we've all heard, the most important. It sets you up both physically and mentally for whatever life might throw at you.

After all, healthy food to our bodies is the same as good-quality fuel to a car; without it we're going to stall, break down and make some very grumpy noises! It's so important to start as we intend to go on, and that means no skipping breakfast, no grabbing a sugar-laden croissant from the café on the corner and no instant fix from a Cadbury's bar: I've been there – the after effects aren't nearly as delicious as the chocolate itself.

By now, I'm pretty sure you'll be thinking this is all leading to: 'Just eat a healthy breakfast!' Not exactly; I know it's not that simple. Whether you're a student with a busy schedule, an office worker with a 7 a.m. start or a new parent who's been up all night, finding time in the morning to make yourself a superfood feast just isn't going to happen. And even with all the time in the world, not all of us have wallets that can comply.

When I first started eating healthily, I didn't think it would be possible to create well-balanced, delicious breakfasts both quickly and cheaply. Needless to say, muesli and oat milk were on the menu for a good six months. But eating the same meals every day doesn't inspire a love of healthy food, and I'm pretty sure that if it wasn't for that light bulb moment when I realised I loved cooking and inventing recipes, I'd have been back to a chocolate muffin and Americano in no time.

In discovering how 'healthy' didn't need to be a drag, and could be affordable and attainable to anybody, I've created a whole range of delicious breakfasts, effortless to prepare and which, with a few minor adjustments, should fit seamlessly into your everyday life.

To make the process as easy as possible (because changing your diet is testing at the best of times), I've included 'How To' instructions for some of the basic recipes, both in this chapter and throughout the book, so you can adapt them for using with your favourite foods or the ones you have to hand. These recipes will support you and your body every day. And the best part? No fuss involved.

Baked carrot cake oatmeal

SERVES 4–6

Coconut oil, for greasing
4 carrots, peeled and grated
200g (2 cups) (gluten-free) rolled oats
1½ teaspoons peeled and grated fresh root ginger
1½ teaspoons ground cinnamon
40g (¼ cup) sultanas
80ml (⅓ cup) pure maple syrup
Pinch of salt
600ml (2½ cups) dairy-free milk of your choice (to make your own, see pages 74–75)

Maple pecan topping
3 tablespoons coconut oil
60ml (¼ cup) pure maple syrup
230g (2 cups) pecans

TIP

Be open-minded! While, yes, there is carrot in this recipe, it doesn't taste like grated carrot, I promise!

I'm a big fan of baked oatmeal and this recipe has been my favourite way of making it so far. It's so full of flavour and incredibly comforting at the same time. I love it with a dollop of whipped coconut cream (see page 66).

Preheat the oven to 180°C/160°C fan/gas 4 and grease a baking dish (roughly 20cm x 25cm) with a little coconut oil. Place the grated carrots in a bowl with the oats, ginger, cinnamon, sultanas, maple syrup and salt. Stir well, then add the milk and mix in before pouring the mixture into the prepared baking dish.

Next make the maple pecan topping. Place the coconut oil in a saucepan and melt over a low heat. Remove from the heat and add the maple syrup, then add the pecans and mix together well.

Scatter the maple-coated pecans on top of the oat mixture in the dish before placing in the oven and baking for 25–30 minutes.

HOW TO MAKE A
Smoothie Bowl

Smoothie bowls are the perfect way to pack in lots of goodness first thing in the morning, and, made with the right combination of ingredients, they can be so delicious. Think of them as a much more flavourful, thicker version of a yoghurt. It's honestly the perfect dairy-free alternative. They're incredibly filling, and can be tailored each day to how you're feeling – sweeter, greener, thicker, smoother! You're never limited to what ingredients you can use for these, and this 'How To' section will show you how to get the ideal balance of protein, fruit, greens and liquid for what I would deem to be the perfect smoothie bowl. The rest is up to you! Get your chef hat on for 3 minutes in the morning and you won't be disappointed.

The perfect smoothie bowl is made with ingredients taken from seven categories: Base, Fruit, Greens, Protein, Liquid, Extras (optional) and Toppings (optional). In the lists that follow, I've given you lots of options to choose from, and the right serving for each ingredient. Ingredients highlighted in green are best for green smoothies; those in pink are best for berry smoothies. Those with no highlighting are great in any type of smoothie.

SERVES 1

BASE
You're going to need a mild-tasting creamy fruit to make your base. Choose one of the following:

1 banana, peeled
1 mango, peeled and stoned
½ avocado, peeled and stoned

Note
For those of you who don't like banana, mango or avocado (silly people!), you can use about 25g (¼ cup) rolled oats instead, though you'll need to make sure you have enough sweetness by adding fruit from below.

FRUIT
To add a fruity layer to your creamy base, you need some tangy-tasting fruit. My favourite are berries, but you can choose one or a combination of any of the following:

about 125g (1 cup) blueberries
about 120g (1 cup) raspberries
about 140g (1 cup) mixed berries
1 eating apple, peeled (optional),
    cored and chopped
1 pear, peeled (optional),
    cored and chopped

GREENS
Whatever type of smoothie you're making, greens are great. The quantity will vary according to the smoothie and personal preference; I normally suggest 1–2 handfuls of greens to start with.

Choose from the following:
1 handful of spinach
1 handful of chopped kale (stems removed)
¼ cucumber, peeled and chopped
    (about 75g prepared weight)
2 stalks of celery (about 80g)
1 handful of chopped romaine lettuce
    (about 40g)

PROTEIN
It's so important to get the nutritional balance of your smoothie right. You don't want your blood-sugar levels sky-rocketing; adding protein stabilises the amount of sugar in your blood and gives slow-releasing energy, meaning you'll be sustained, energised and feel fuller for longer. Choose one of the following:

2 tablespoons ground flaxseeds
1 tablespoon nut or seed butter
    (to make your own, see page 58)
30g (¼ cup) nuts (my favourite for smoothies
    are cashews, though you can also use brazil
    nuts, almonds or pecans), soaked for at
    least 2 hours or overnight, then drained
30g brown rice protein powder
30g hemp protein powder

LIQUID

For a smoothie you only need a minimal amount of liquid to let the mixture blend properly. This ranges between 60ml to 120ml (¼ to ½ cup). Start with the former and work up; don't hesitate to add more if your blender is struggling to blend everything – some models are more high-powered than others. Choose one of the following:

Almond milk
Rice milk
Full-fat coconut milk or water
Freshly squeezed orange juice
Water

EXTRAS (OPTIONAL)

There are lots of great extras you can add to your smoothie bowl – by no means essential, but great for you. Whether it's a superfood to boost your health or a sweetener to satisfy your sweet tooth, here are my favourites. Feel free to add however many/few you like.

1 tablespoon chia seeds
2 tablespoons (gluten-free) rolled oats
1–2 Medjool dates, pitted and chopped
1 teaspoon baobab powder
1 teaspoon maca powder
2 teaspoons acai berry powder
1 teaspoon spirulina powder
1 teaspoon wheatgrass powder
1 teaspoon chlorella powder
1 teaspoon green complex powder
    (a mixture of the superfood greens)

TOPPINGS (OPTIONAL)

This is a little sprinkle of goodness that you can add to the top of the smoothie bowl, if you like, for a bit of crunch. The combination of smooth and crunchy is to die for. Add a sprinkling of one of the following:

Granola (try my Golden Granola on page 66)
Muesli (try my my Flax and Goji Berry Muesli
    on page 65)
Cacao nibs
Desiccated coconut
Trail mix (try my version on page 171)

METHOD

The method couldn't be simpler: just add something (or a combination of things) from each category into your blender (it may need to be a high-powered blender or a food processor if you're including nuts) and blend!

Tip
I hate washing up; it's the last thing I want to do early in the morning. To prepare a smoothie bowl, you only use a blender, a bowl, spoon and perhaps a vegetable knife, but to further cut down on the washing-up after smoothie-making, just add a squirt of washing-up liquid and some hot water to the blender and blend again. This will get rid of any smoothie left in the blender, and then all you need to do is rinse. Simples!

Get-up-and-glow green smoothie bowl

SERVES 1

½ avocado, peeled and stoned
1 pear, cored and chopped
1 handful of spinach
1 handful of chopped kale
    (stems removed)
1 tablespoon almond butter
80ml (⅓ cup) almond milk
1 teaspoon spirulina powder
    (optional)
Golden granola, for topping
    (see page 66 – optional)

TIP

Make sure the kale and
spinach are well washed,
even if they're the most
organic of greens. You
don't want any unwanted
bacteria or pesticides in
your smoothie – definitely
not a desirable 'extra'!

This smoothie bowl is brimming with nutrients, and contains what I would class as the ultimate balance of healthy fats, chlorophyll-rich greens and plant-based protein, giving you a steady flow of energy all morning. Although this smoothie is green, it has an amazing sweetness, and is truly delicious despite its not so appealing colour.

Simply blend all the ingredients except the topping in your blender until smooth. Pour into a bowl, add a sprinkling of Golden granola, if you like, and enjoy!

Opposite, clockwise from top: Super-berry bowl, Golden granola, Berry-creamy smoothie bowl, Get-up-and-glow green smoothie bowl

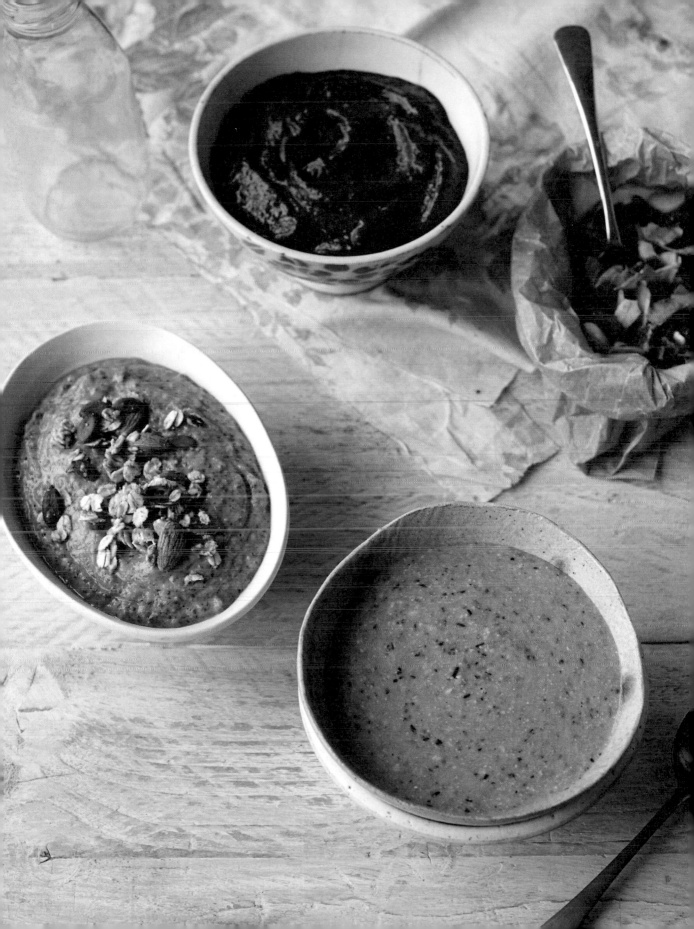

Berry-creamy smoothie bowl

SERVES 1

1 banana, peeled, sliced
    and frozen
60g (½ cup) blueberries
60g (½ cup) raspberries
30g (¼ cup) raw cashews,
    soaked in water for at least
    2 hours or overnight,
    then drained
120ml (½ cup) dairy-free
    milk of your choice
    (to make your own,
    see pages 74–75)
1 tablespoon chia seeds
    (optional)
Topping of your choice
    from the 'How To' list
    (see page 31 – optional)

This is one of my favourite smoothie bowls, and the recipe I play around with all the time. The cashews provide the most incredible creaminess and really help to thicken the smoothie. As well as adding texture, they're also packed with nutrients. (See photo on page 33).

◇◇◇◇◇◇◇◇◇◇◇◇◇◇◇◇◇◇◇◇◇◇◇◇◇◇◇◇

Add everything to your blender and blend! Pour into a bowl and, if you like, add the topping of your choice.

SWITCH IT UP

Blueberries and raspberries work well in this recipe, but you can use blackberries, strawberries or pomegranate seeds, and it will be just as tasty and nutritious. If you don't want to include banana in this recipe, you can substitute it with 25g (¼ cup) (gluten-free) rolled oats. You can also try adding a couple of pitted Medjool dates or an extra 75g (½ cup) of berries.

Super-berry bowl

1 banana, peeled, sliced
   and frozen
150g (1 cup) frozen berries
   (blueberries and
   raspberries are best)
1 tablespoon ground
   flaxseeds
60ml (¼ cup) freshly
   squeezed orange juice
2 teaspoons acai berry
   powder (optional)
Trail Mix, for topping
   (optional – see page 171)

TIP

If you don't have acai berry
powder, no sweat – you can
use any superfood powder
or none at all. The smoothie
will still be delicious and
very good for you.

This was my first introduction to smoothie bowls, and the reason I fell in love with them. It's a little bit different from a normal smoothie, however. As the fruit is frozen, the consistency is more like that of an ice cream – brilliant for those warm summer mornings. (See photo on page 33).

Add all the ingredients except the topping to your blender and blend! If your blender isn't very high-powered, you may need to add a little more fresh orange juice or water to help purée the frozen fruit. Alternatively, blend everything in a food processor. Top with my Trail Mix, if you like.

Chickpea 'crêpe' with tomatoes and mushrooms

SERVES 1

1–2 tablespoons olive oil
150g (1½ cups) sliced
    white mushrooms
225g (1½ cups) cherry
    tomatoes, halved
75g (⅓ cup) passata
½ avocado, peeled,
    stoned and sliced

'Crêpe' batter
25g (¼ cup) chickpea flour
    (besan or gram flour)
1 tablespoon nutritional
    yeast (optional)
60ml (¼ cup) plus 2
    tablespoons water
1 tablespoon finely chopped
    chives or red onion
Salt and pepper

TIP

If you can't be bothered to wash up two pans, use the same frying pan for both parts of the recipe. Make the crêpe first, and keep it in the oven to stay warm while you cook the tomatoes and mushrooms.

This crêpe doesn't taste like a conventional one made with eggs, but it is completely delicious in its own right. It's perfect for a savoury breakfast and is incredibly filling. The 'crêpe' wrap is made with chickpea flour, which has the benefit of being inexpensive and a great investment as you tend to use only small quantities of it.

◇◇◇◇◇◇◇◇◇◇◇◇◇◇◇◇◇◇◇◇◇◇◇◇◇◇◇◇◇◇◇◇

Start by combining all the ingredients for the crêpe batter in a bowl, season with a pinch of salt and a little pepper and whisk until smooth – just as you would for an crêpe made with eggs.

Add the olive oil to a frying pan. When the oil is hot, add the mushrooms and cherry tomatoes. Sauté over a medium heat for about 4 minutes until the mushrooms are browned and the tomatoes softened. Add the passata and bring to the boil, then reduce the heat to low and cover with a lid to keep warm while you make the chickpea crêpe.

Add a little olive oil to a 22cm-diameter frying pan over a high heat and then pour in the crêpe batter, tipping the mixture around the pan to form a very thin, even layer. Cook for around 3 minutes on one side, carefully flip over with a spatula and cook for another 3 minutes on the other side.

Tip the crêpe onto your plate, pour over the mushroom and tomato mixture and top with the avocado before folding over and enjoying.

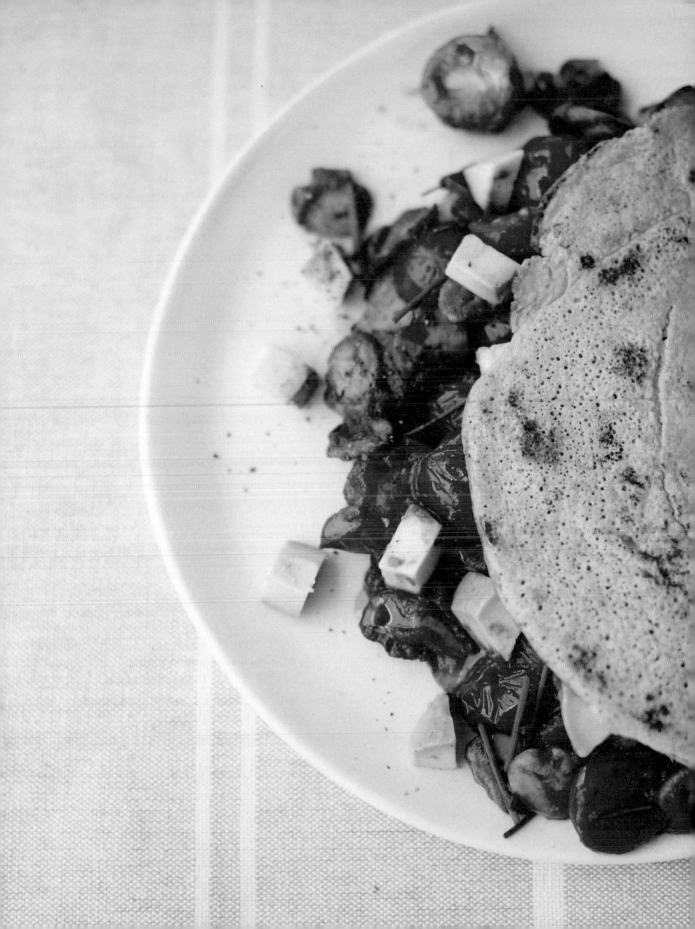

HOW TO MAKE A

Power-packed Bowl of porridge

Porridge may be regarded as the classic 'healthy' breakfast, but personally I think it can be incredibly bland and actually not that nutritious. While oats are full of fibre and very easy to cook, it's important to have a range of nutrients to start the day. This 'How To' section shows you how to build a goodness-packed bowl that is both cost effective and keeps you energised and satisfied all morning – the formula for one amazing bowl of porridge!

SERVES 1

DAIRY-FREE MILK
Choose one of the following (or make your own – see pages 74–75):
350ml (1½ cups) almond milk
350ml (1½ cups) full-fat coconut milk
350ml (1½ cups) rice milk
350ml (1½ cups) oat milk
240ml (1 cup) water plus 120ml (½ cup) tinned full-fat coconut milk

GRAIN
Choose one of the following:
50g (½ cup) (gluten-free) rolled oats (my favourite!)
85g (½ cup) buckwheat
50g (½ cup) quinoa flakes

FRUIT
Choose 1–3 of the following:
1 banana, peeled and sliced or mashed
40g (⅓ cup) blueberries
40g (⅓ cup) raspberries
45g (¼ cup) pomegranate seeds
1 eating apple, peeled (optional), cored and cubed
1 pear, peeled (optional), cored and sliced
2 Medjool dates, pitted and chopped

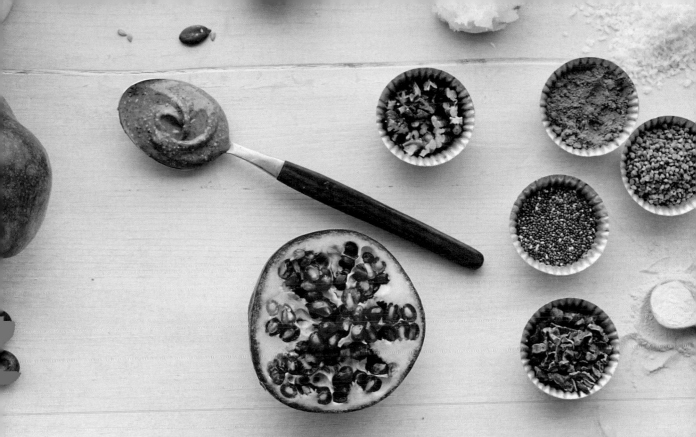

PROTEIN

Choose 1–3 of the following:

2 tablespoons ground flaxseeds

1 tablespoon nut/seed butter
    (to make your own, see page 58)

1 handful of crushed nuts (cashews, pecans,
    almonds, hazelnuts or walnuts), for sprinkling

1–2 tablespoons seeds (flaxseeds, sunflower
    or pumpkin seeds), for sprinkling

EXTRAS (OPTIONAL)

Choose none or all of them – go wild!

1 teaspoon ground cinnamon

1 teaspoon ground ginger

1–2 tablespoons raw cacao (or cocoa) powder

1 teaspoon bee pollen

1 teaspoon baobab powder

1 tablespoon chia seeds

2 tablespoons desiccated coconut

2–4 tablespoons tinned coconut cream
    (or you could use my homemade
    sweet cream – see page 66)

1 tablespoon coconut oil, melted

1 teaspoon raw honey, agave or pure maple syrup

METHOD

1 Pick your milk and pour into a pan set over
a medium-high heat. When the milk starts to
bubble, add your grain of choice and lower
the heat to a simmer.

2 At this point, wash and prepare your fruit
and add to the pan if you want it to melt into
the porridge; if not, stir it into the porridge when
it's cooked. Keep on stirring and add any spices
or supplements (cinnamon, ginger, cacao/cocoa
powder, bee pollen, baobab powder, chia seeds).

3 Once the porridge is cooked through – after
simmering for 5-10 minutes – add your choice
of protein (if using ground flaxseeds or nut/
seed butter) and pour into a bowl. Top with any
extra fruit, a sprinkling of seeds, crushed nuts or
desiccated coconut and a drizzle of coconut oil
or raw honey, agave or maple syrup if you wish!

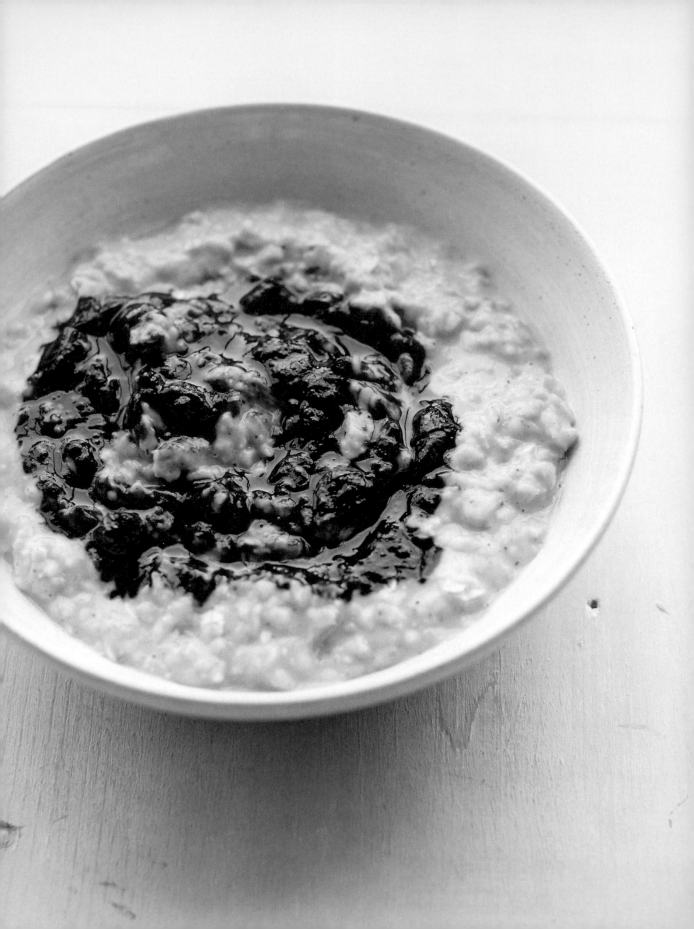

Almond, cinnamon and banana porridge with a blueberry compote

SERVES 1

350ml (1½ cups) almond milk
50g (½ cup) (gluten-free) rolled oats
1 banana
¼ teaspoon ground cinnamon (optional)
1 tablespoon almond butter

Blueberry compote
60g (½ cup) blueberries
1 tablespoon water
1 teaspoon fresh lemon juice

TIP
You can make the blueberry compote just after you've poured out the porridge, using the same pan to save on washing-up.

This porridge combines some classic flavours: the gentle spiciness of the cinnamon; the nuttiness of the almond milk; and the intense burst of sweetness from the banana and blueberries. Wonderfully rich and completely moreish, this is an everyday staple in my household!

Pour the almond milk into a pan set over a medium-high heat. When it starts to bubble, add the oats and lower the heat to a simmer.

Peel and mash the banana and add to the pan if you want it to melt into the porridge; if not, stir it into the porridge when it's cooked. Add the cinnamon, if using, and simmer for 5–10 minutes, stirring frequently.

Just before the porridge is ready, make the compote. Pop the blueberries, water and lemon juice into a small pan set over a high heat. Get the blueberries bubbling away before gently pushing them down and bursting them with your wooden spoon. When it becomes a smooth compote with a few whole plump blueberries remaining, remove from the heat.

Once the porridge is cooked through, stir in the almond butter and pour into your bowl, spoon over the compote and enjoy!

SWITCH IT UP
Blueberries make a delicious compote and go so well with the banana and cinnamon, but you can also use raspberries, strawberries or blackberries instead.

Coconut and raspberry porridge

SERVES 1

240ml (1 cup) water plus
120ml (½ cup) tinned
full-fat coconut milk

50g (½ cup) (gluten-free)
rolled oats

60–90g (½–¾ cup)
raspberries

½ teaspoon pure vanilla
extract

1 tablespoon raw honey,
agave or pure maple syrup
(optional – for sweetening)

1 handful of crushed cashews,
for sprinkling

Coconut and raspberry are a match made in heaven – I'm constantly using this combination to make the most satisfying and delicious breakfasts and desserts. All the ingredients here are pantry staples – oats, coconut milk, raw honey, vanilla extract and cashew nuts – with the exception of the raspberries, which I buy fresh each week, though you could of course use frozen berries. If raspberries aren't available, or you're not a big fan, I've suggested a couple of great alternatives below for switching it up!

Pour the water into a pan set over a medium-high heat. When it starts to bubble, add the oats and lower the heat to a simmer.

Add the coconut milk and tip in the raspberries if you want them to melt into the porridge; if not, stir them into the porridge when it's cooked. Add the vanilla extract and simmer for 5–10 minutes, stirring frequently.

When cooked, stir in the honey or syrup (if needed) before pouring into your bowl and sprinkling with the crushed cashews.

SWITCH IT UP

Raspberries and coconut are an incredible combo, but why not try blueberries or banana instead of the raspberries? Yum!

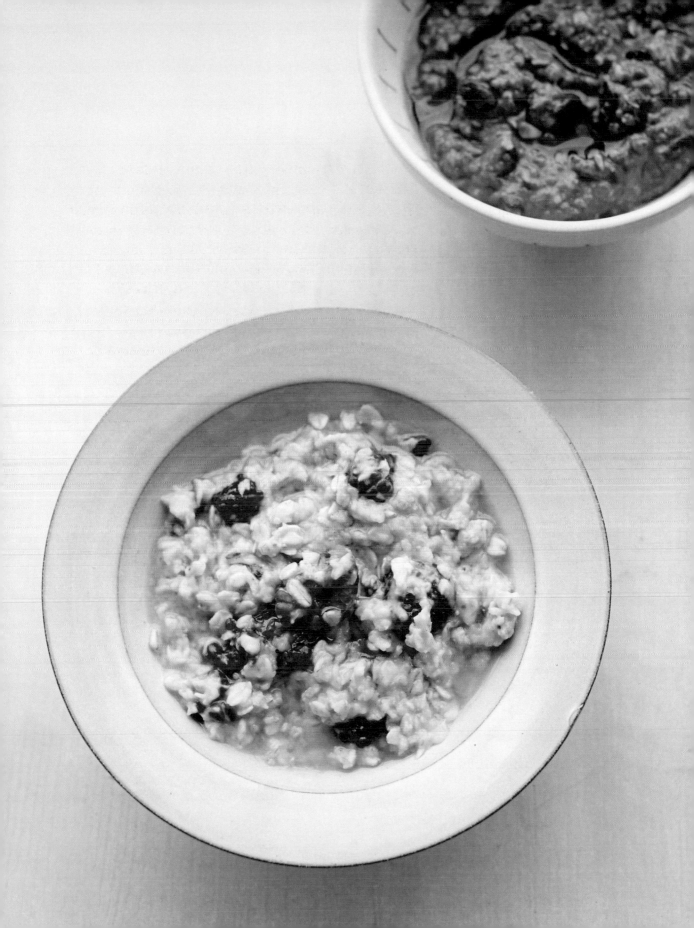

Chocolate porridge

350ml (1½ cups) rice milk, plus extra if needed
50g (½ cup) (gluten-free) rolled oats
1 banana
1 tablespoon raw cacao (or cocoa) powder
1 handful of dried goji berries (optional)
1 tablespoon almond butter
½–1 tablespoon pure maple syrup (optional – for sweetening if the almond milk is very bitter)

If you're a chocoholic like me, a bowl of this porridge is the most amazing way to satisfy your chocolate cravings first thing! While 'chocolate' is indeed in the name, I don't use any refined sugars or dairy products in this recipe. The ingredients I do use – banana, rice milk and almond butter – all help to intensify the chocolate flavour of the cacao (or cocoa) powder, but in a completely natural way. (See photo on page 43).

Pour the rice milk into a pan set over a medium-high heat. When it starts to bubble, add the oats and lower the heat to a simmer.

Peel and mash the banana and add to the pan if you want it to melt into the porridge; if not, stir it into the porridge when it's cooked. Add the cacao (or cocoa) powder and goji berries (if using) and simmer for 5–10 minutes, stirring frequently and adding up to 120ml (½ cup) more milk if needed.

When cooked, stir in the almond butter and the maple syrup (if needed), pour into a bowl and serve with any fresh berries you like!

Banoffee overnight oats

SERVES 1

50g (½ cup) (gluten-free)
    rolled oats
240ml (1 cup) almond
    or rice milk
1 banana, peeled
1 tablespoon almond butter

½ teaspoon ground cinnamon
2 Medjool dates, pitted
    and chopped

This recipe is so easy, and tastes fabulous – like a fusion of banana, caramel and almonds. It's the best breakfast for a busy morning and a real winner with everyone: I can never get away with making just a single portion and end up preparing big batches for both me and my flatmates. (See photo on page 49).

◇◇◇◇◇◇◇◇◇◇◇◇◇◇◇◇◇◇◇◇◇◇◇◇◇◇◇◇◇◇◇◇◇◇◇◇◇

Start by mixing the oats and milk together in a bowl. Mash the banana and almond butter together until smooth, then add to the oat mixture with the cinnamon and chopped dates.

Mix well and pour into a clean jar (or leave in the bowl if you're eating in). Top with blueberries or any other fruit you like, pop the lid on the jar (or cover the bowl) and store in the fridge overnight.

HOW TO MAKE

Overnight Oats

Anyone who comes to stay with me will always find a jar of oaty goodness in my fridge. This jar is my saviour when it comes to busy mornings – Overnight Oats are my answer to keeping healthy on the go. They take no time at all to make the night before (3–10 minutes, depending on how fancy you want to them to be) and in the morning are the perfect 'grab and go'. All you need is a spoon! They're also great to make in big batches (without the fresh fruit) as they last in the fridge for about 5 days without going off. I sometimes spend 10 minutes on a Sunday evening preparing the recipe for one multiplied by five in a big bowl and pouring it into an airtight container, from which I decant a single serving, adding the fresh fruit and a little extra milk, if needed, the night before, all ready for the following day. Here's my 'How To' for assembling a perfectly balanced jar or bowl of Overnight Oats.

SERVES 1

GRAIN
50g (½ cup) (gluten-free) rolled oats

DAIRY-FREE MILK
Choose 1 of the following (or make your own – see pages 74–75):
350ml (1½ cups) almond milk
350ml (1½ cups) full-fat coconut milk
350ml (1½ cups) rice milk
350ml (1½ cups) oat milk

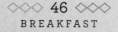

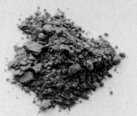

FRUIT

Choose 1–3 of the following:
1 banana, peeled and sliced
40g (⅓ cup) blueberries
40g (⅓ cup) raspberries
45g (¼ cup) pomegranate seeds
½ mango, peeled, stoned and sliced
1 eating apple, peeled (optional),
    cored and cubed
1 pear, peeled (optional), cored and sliced
1–2 Medjool dates, pitted and chopped

EXTRAS (OPTIONAL)

Choose as many (or few) as you like!
1 tablespoon raw cacao (or cocoa) powder
1 tablespoon almond butter
½ teaspoon vanilla extract
1 tablespoon chia seeds
1 tablespoon pumpkin seeds
2 tablespoons ground flaxseeds
2 tablespoons desiccated coconut
2 tablespoons dried goji berries
1 tablespoon cacao nibs

ADDITIONS (OPTIONAL)

Choose one of the following:
4 tablespoons mango-cashew cream
    (see page 50)
4 tablespoons Raspberry and chia jam
    (see page 57)
4 tablespoons Apricot jam (see page 57)
4 tablespoons Apple and ginger compote
    (see page 51)

METHOD

1 Start by mixing the oats and milk together in a bowl. If using any extras, stir them in them now, then pour the mixture into a clean jar with a lid (this is great if you're taking the oats to go) or leave in the bowl (if you're eating in).

2 If you want to include any additions – the mango-cashew cream or the compote, for instance, or one of the jams – pour these on top of the oat mixture in the jar/bowl.

3 Prepare your choice of fruit and simply throw on top of the oat mixture, or, if you like, you can get fancy and layer it between the oats. Put the lid on the jar (or cover the bowl) and store in the fridge overnight.

Chocolate overnight oats with crushed raspberries and coconut

SERVES 1

50g (½ cup) (gluten-free) rolled oats
240ml (1 cup) rice milk
1 tablespoon chia seeds
1 tablespoon cacao (or cocoa) powder (or to taste)
1 banana, peeled and mashed
40g (⅓ cup) raspberries, crushed
2 tablespoons desiccated coconut, for sprinkling

TIP

If you can't find rice milk, you can use any other dairy-free milk from the 'How To' list (see page 46). Add a teaspoon of raw honey, agave or pure maple syrup to offset any bitterness from the milk or cacao powder. Alternatively, just add a little less cacao powder!

Including raw cacao (or cocoa) powder in your Overnight Oats is an easy way to add an extra dimension to your wake-me up meal. Wonderfully rich in flavour, it makes the oat mixture taste more sustaining than a regular bowlful, keeping you full and energised all morning.

◇◇◇◇◇◇◇◇◇◇◇◇◇◇◇◇◇◇◇◇◇◇◇◇◇◇◇◇◇◇◇◇◇◇

Start by mixing the oats and milk together in a bowl. Add the chia seeds, cacao (or cocoa) powder and mashed banana and mix until everything is combined and already tasting completely delicious.

Now all you have to do is pour the mixture into a clean jar (or just leave the mixture in the bowl if you're eating in) and top with the crushed raspberries and a sprinkling of desiccated coconut. Screw the lid on the jar (or cover the bowl) and leave in the fridge overnight.

SWITCH IT UP

Pomegranate seeds would work very well in this recipe as an alternative to the raspberries.

Opposite, clockwise from top left: Apple and ginger overnight oats, Mango and cashew overnight oats (with pumpkin seeds), Chocolate overnight oats with crushed raspberries and coconut, Banoffee overnight oats.

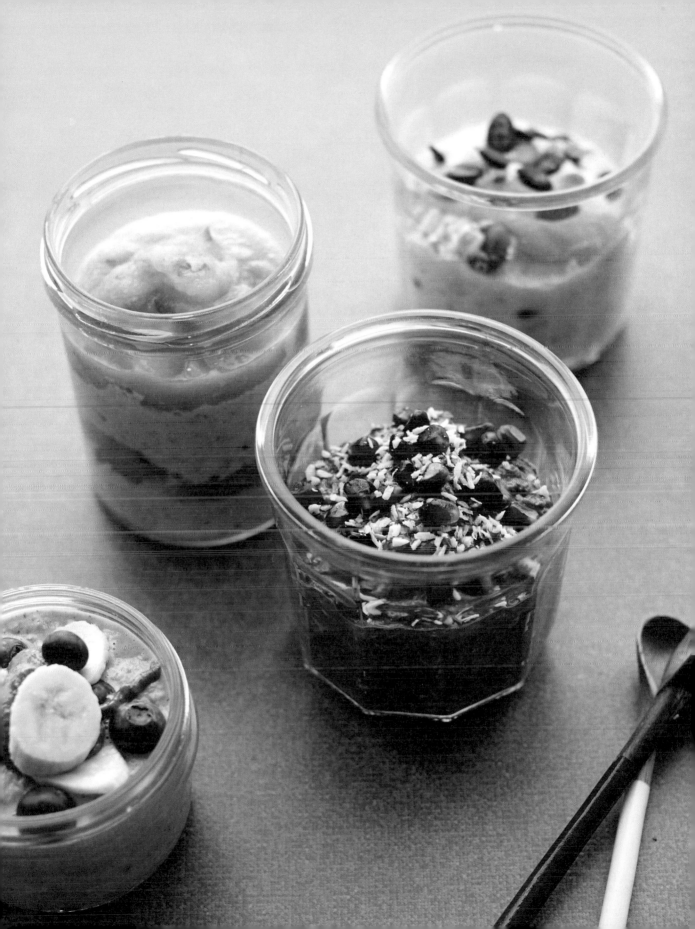

Mango and cashew overnight oats

SERVES 1

50g (½ cup) (gluten-free)
    rolled oats
240ml (1 cup) dairy-free milk
    of your choice (to make
    your own, see pages 74–75)
1 tablespoon chia seeds
30g (¼ cup) blueberries
1 tablespoon pumpkin seeds,
    for sprinkling

**Mango-cashew cream
(makes enough for
2 portions!)**
1 mango, peeled and stoned
30g (¼ cup) raw cashews,
    soaked in water for at
    least 2 hours or overnight,
    then drained
2–4 tablespoons dairy-
    free milk (to help the
    mixture blend)

TIP

Make a big batch of the
mango-cashew cream at the
weekend. As well as using
it in this recipe, you can pair
it with my Golden Granola
(as an alternative to the
coconut cream there – see
page 66) or some fresh fruit
and take it 'to go' as an
afternoon pick-me-up.

OK, so this recipe isn't quite as simple as the
others – there is a little blending involved –
but, trust me, it's absolutely worth it. The mango-
cashew cream makes more than you need for
a single portion, so you can make this recipe
two days running for maximum indulgence!
(See photo on page 49).

Mix the oats and milk together in a bowl and add
the chia seeds and blueberries. Mix everything
together well and place in a clean jar (or leave in
the bowl for eating in).

To make the mango-cashew cream, chop up the
mango and blend with the cashews and enough
milk to form a cream. Add to the oat mixture and
scatter with the pumpkin seeds. Screw the lid on
the jar (or cover the bowl) and pop in the fridge
to chill overnight.

Apple and ginger overnight oats

SERVES 1

50g (½ cup) (gluten-free)
    rolled oats
240ml (1 cup) dairy-free milk
    of your choice (to make
    your own, see pages 74–75)
1 tablespoon chia seeds

**Apple and ginger compote
(makes a jarful)**
250g (1 cup) apple purée
90g (½ cup) Medjool dates,
    pitted and chopped
1 teaspoon peeled and finely
    chopped fresh root ginger
¼ teaspoon ground cinnamon

Apple, ginger and cinnamon are a combination to be reckoned with and, paired with the subtly nutty flavour of the oats, you've got yourself a truly delicious breakfast. (See photo on page 49).

First make the apple and ginger compote by mixing together all the ingredients for the compote. Place in a clean jam jar or airtight plastic container and store in the fridge (where it will last for up to a week).

Mix the oats and milk together in a bowl and stir in the chia seeds. Layer with about 80g (⅓ cup) of the apple and ginger compote – either in a jar or another bowl – then cover and store overnight in the fridge for a delicious breakfast at home or on the go.

Coconut chia pudding with crushed raspberries

SERVES 2

15g (¼ cup) unsweetened shredded coconut

40g (¼ cup) chia seeds

180ml (¾ cup) full-fat coconut milk

120ml (½ cup) coconut water

1 teaspoon pure vanilla extract

60g (½ cup) raspberries, crushed

Like Overnight Oats (see pages 46–47), this is another dish that you can prepare the night before to ensure you have a great breakfast waiting for you first thing in the morning – really delicious and no fuss involved. Just like Overnight Oats, you can make a big batch of this and it keeps really well in the fridge. If I have a really busy week ahead, I'll make enough for every day, whether it's for snacking or breakfast on the go.

◇◇◇◇◇◇◇◇◇◇◇◇◇◇◇◇◇◇◇◇◇◇◇◇◇◇◇◇◇◇

In a small bowl or jar, combine all the ingredients except the raspberries and mix well. Spoon the raspberries on top, then cover and leave in the fridge overnight.

SWITCH IT UP

This dish is also incredible topped with sliced banana or a sprinkling of pomegranate seeds.

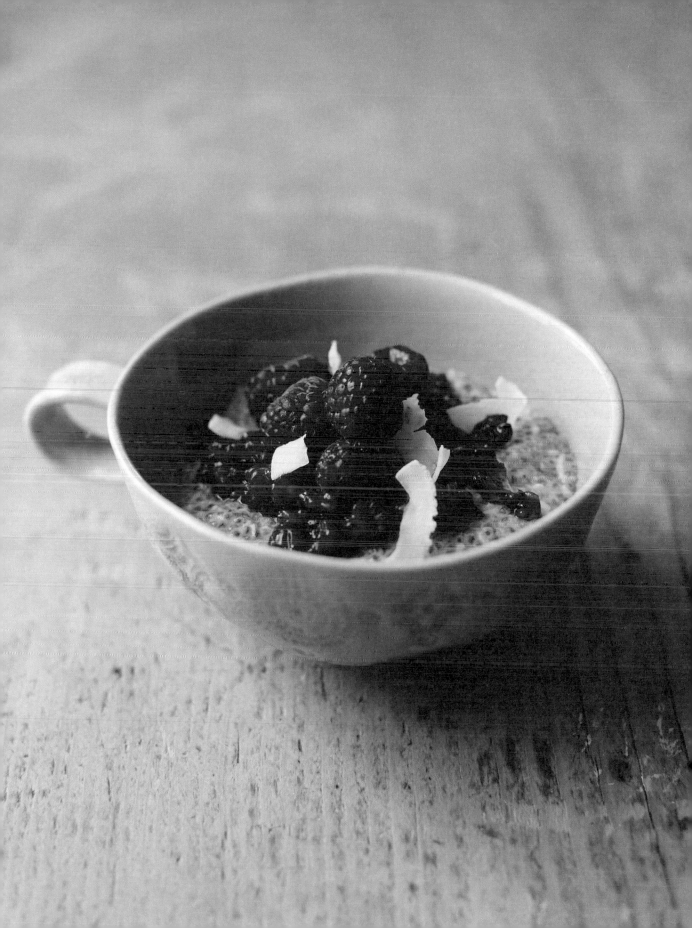

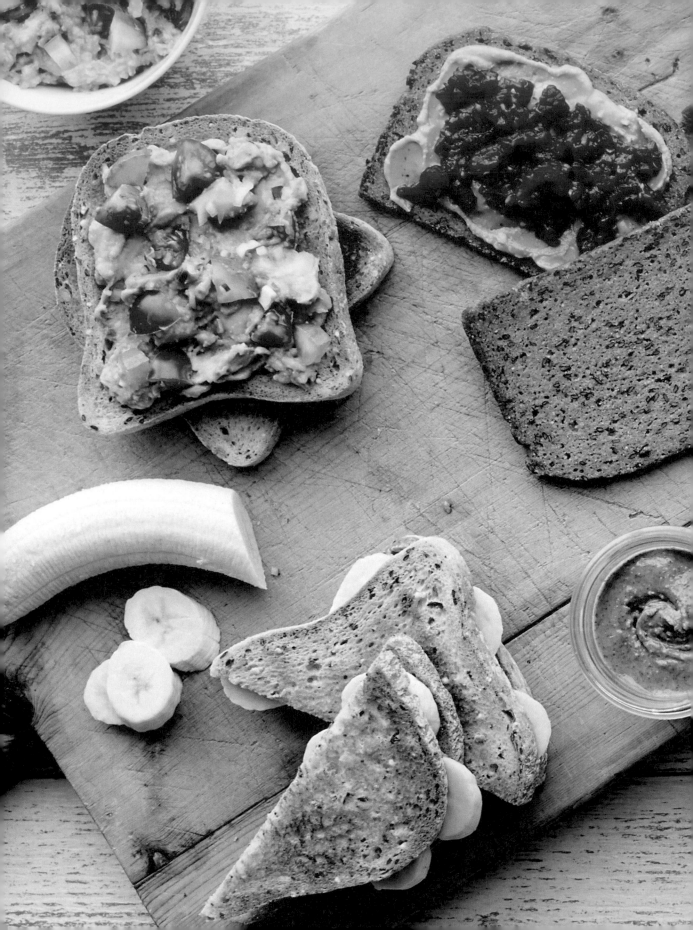

The on-the-go breakfast sandwiches

I'm a big toast fan and often use these On-the-go Breakfast Sandwich mixtures spread on gluten-free toast (made, for instance, with my Quinoa and chia bread – see page 63) to eat at home, but they are excellent, too, as fillings for fresh sandwiches on the go. They're dead-easy, dead-tasty combinations that anyone, from my baby nephew to my grandma, would enjoy. And like Overnight oats (see pages 46–47), you can make them the night before: simply wrap them in foil and pop them in the fridge overnight to enjoy for breakfast or brunch when you're out and about.

Almond butter and banana

MAKES 1 SANDWICH

2 slices of gluten-free bread
2–4 generous tablespoons almond butter
½ large banana, peeled and sliced

Simply spread each slice of bread with the almond butter, top one piece with the sliced banana and sandwich together with the other piece of bread.

Sassy's peanut butter and 'jelly' sandwich

MAKES 1 SANDWICH

2 slices of gluten-free bread
2–4 generous tablespoons peanut butter
120g (1 cup) raspberries, crushed

Simply spread each slice of bread with the peanut butter, top one piece with the crushed raspberries and sandwich together with the other piece of bread. Amazing!

Avocado, tomato, onion and lemon

MAKES 1 SANDWICH

2 slices of gluten-free bread
½ avocado, peeled and stoned
Juice of ½ lemon
¼ red onion (about 40g), peeled and finely chopped
75g (½ cup) cherry tomatoes, quartered
¼ cucumber, peeled and finely chopped
2 slices of gluten-free bread

Place the avocado and lemon juice in a bowl and mash together until smooth. Mix in the onion, tomatoes and cucumber. Spread the mixture onto one of the slices of bread, top with the other piece of bread and voilà!

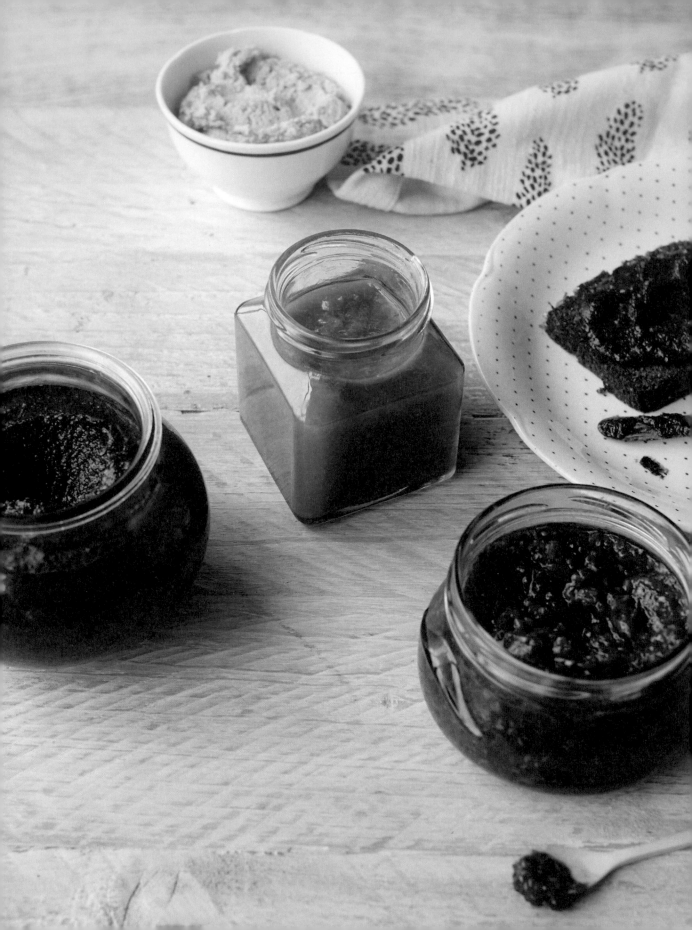

Spreads

I love jam and Nutella, so these healthier versions of standard spreads are important staples in my kitchen. They're so easy to make, too, and require only a few ingredients. As they're made from entirely natural ingredients and contain no preservatives, make sure you store them in a jar or other airtight container in the fridge.

Apricot jam

MAKES 1 JAR

8 fresh apricots
4 tablespoons water
2 tablespoons raw honey,
    agave or pure maple syrup
Juice of 1 lemon

Pit and quarter the apricots – don't bother peeling them. Add to a pan with the water, honey or agave/maple syrup and lemon juice. Bring to the boil, then reduce the heat and simmer for about 10 minutes, stirring all the while, until reduced but still slightly runny. (The jam will thicken when it cools.)

Transfer to a clean jam jar or airtight plastic container, cover with a lid and leave to cool before storing in the fridge for up to 8 days.

Raspberry and chia jam

MAKES 1 JAR

120g (1 cup) raspberries
½ eating apple, peeled,
    cored and roughly chopped
2 tablespoons water
1 Medjool date, pitted
1 tablespoon chia seeds
1 tablespoon agave syrup
    or raw honey (optional)

Place the raspberries, apple and water in a blender and blend until smooth. Add the date and chia seeds and blend again.

Transfer to a pan on a medium-high heat and add the agave syrup or honey (if using). Stir the mixture until it starts to boil and caramelise, then pour into a clean jam jar or airtight plastic container, cover with a lid and leave to cool. Store in the fridge until you're ready to use it. (Kept like this, it will last for up to 7 days.)

Opposite, clockwise from top: Nut butter, Apricot jam, Raspberry and chia jam, Raw chocolate and hazelnut spread.

Raw chocolate and hazelnut spread

MAKES 1 JAR

300g (2 cups) blanched hazelnuts
60ml (¼ cup) pure maple syrup
3 tablespoons raw cacao (or cocoa) powder
120ml (½ cup) water

Preheat the oven to 190°C/170°C fan/ gas 5. Spread the hazelnuts out on a baking tray and toast in the oven for around 5 minutes or until golden brown, shaking the tin once or twice to ensure they brown evenly and don't burn. Remove from the oven and allow to cool before placing in a food processor to blend for about 10 minutes, until very finely ground.

Add the maple syrup, cacao (or cocoa) powder, and water and continue to blend until smooth. Transfer to a clean jam jar or airtight plastic container and store in the fridge for up to 7 days.

(Both recipes photographed on page 56)

Nut butter

MAKES 1 JAR

260g (2 cups) nuts of your choice
(my favourites are almonds,
cashews or peanuts)

Preheat the oven to 190°C/170°C fan/ gas 5. Spread the nuts out on a baking tray and pop in the oven for 5–10 minutes until golden brown, shaking once or twice to ensure they brown evenly and don't burn. Remove from the oven and allow to cool down slightly.

Now add to a food processor (the more powerful your machine, the easier it will blend) and process for 10–15 minutes, or until totally smooth. And voilà – homemade nut butter!

Banana pancakes with a blueberry syrup

SERVES 2/
MAKES 6 PANCAKES

100g (1 cup) (gluten-free)
    rolled oats
2–3 Medjool dates,
    pitted and chopped
240–350ml (1–1½ cups)
    dairy-free milk of your
    choice (to make your
    own, see pages 74–75)
1 banana, peeled
40g (⅓ cup) brown rice
    flour
3–4 tablespoons coconut oil

Blueberry syrup
125g (1 cup) blueberries
1 tablespoon water

Everyone loves a good pancake and this recipe has been a favourite of mine for years. Brimming with fibre, vitamins and minerals, these gluten-free pancakes are really satisfying. Instead of giving you that bloated sensation and energy slump you'd normally experience after a pancake feast, they leave you feeling just right, fuelled with an abundance of long-lasting energy.

Start by grinding the oats into a flour-like consistency in a blender, food processor or coffee grinder, then set to one side. Add the dates and milk to the blender or food processor and blend until the date pieces have been obliterated into tiny fragments. Break up the banana into smaller pieces and add to the blender with the brown rice flour. Blend until the mixture is thick and smooth, then pour into a measuring jug.

Add a little coconut oil to a frying pan over a medium heat and allow it to melt before pouring 120ml (½ cup) batter into the pan, spreading it out with a knife into an even circle. You want to make a small pancake, so don't worry if it's quite thick. Cook on one side for roughly 2 minutes, then carefully flip over with a spatula and cook for 2 minutes on the other side. Repeat with the rest of the mixture, adding extra coconut oil as needed and transferring each pancake to a plate as you make it. Keep the stack of pancakes warm in the oven.

Recipe continues overleaf

Recipe continued

Meanwhile, make the blueberry syrup. Simple add the blueberries and water to a saucepan, bring to the boil and allow to bubble away, pushing the blueberries down gently and bursting them with your wooden spoon, until a syrup forms. Stir occasionally to make sure the mixture doesn't catch on the bottom of the pan.

Remove the pan from the heat and drizzle the syrup over the pancakes to serve. They're also amazing served with a dollop of my whipped coconut cream (see page 66).

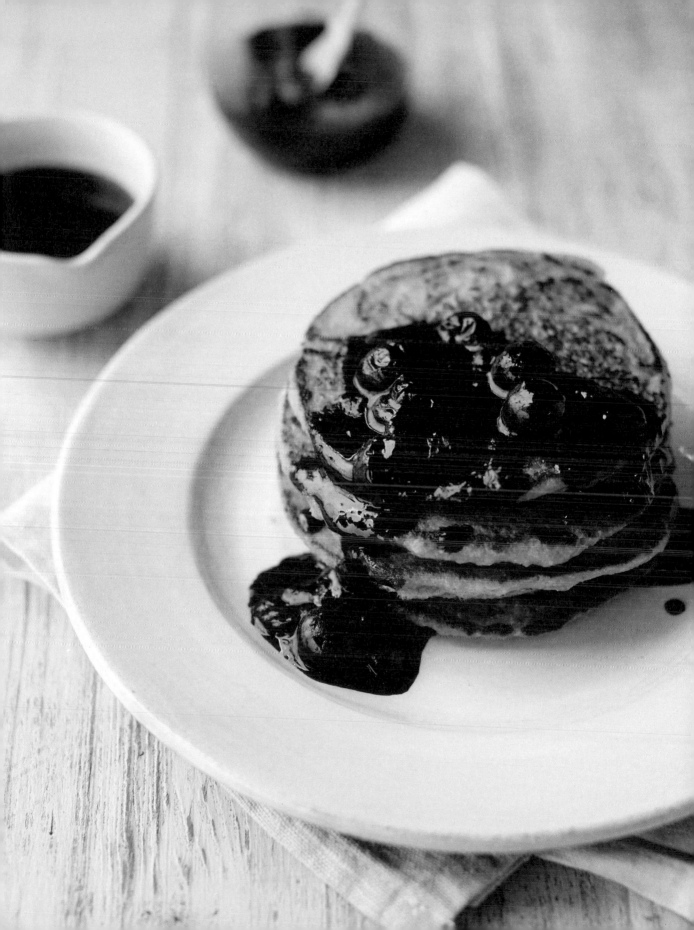

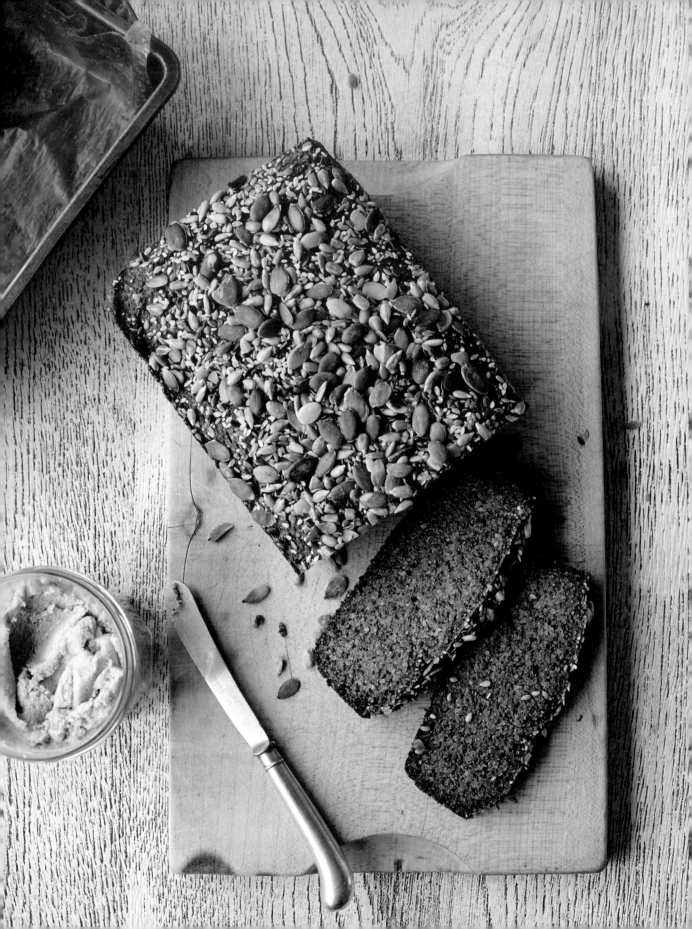

Quinoa and chia bread

MAKES 1 LOAF

340g (2 cups) quinoa
120g (¾ cup) chia seeds
240ml (1 cup) water
60ml (¼ cup) extra-virgin
  olive oil, plus extra
  for greasing
1 teaspoon bicarbonate
  of soda
1 teaspoon raw honey
  or pure maple syrup
3 tablespoons fresh lemon
  juice
Generous pinch of salt
70g (½ cup) mixed seeds,
  for sprinkling

This gluten-free bread has a very different texture to regular bread, but it's ideal for anyone who doesn't have a bread maker and wants an easy recipe for a loaf to eat over the next few days. It's best either toasted, or sliced and baked in the oven. It can be frozen, too, which is great if you want to bake a batch.

The night before you plan on baking the bread, you need to soak the quinoa and chia seeds. Place each in separate bowls, then pour the 240ml/1 cup water over the chia seeds and enough water over the quinoa to cover well. Place both bowls in the fridge to soak overnight.

When you're ready to bake, preheat the oven to 160°C/140°C fan/gas 3, then grease a 450g loaf tin with olive oil and line with baking parchment. Drain the quinoa, then place half the quinoa in a blender with the chia seeds, bicarbonate of soda, honey or maple syrup, olive oil and lemon juice. Blend until the mixture is almost smooth, then stir in the other half of the quinoa.

Pour the mixture into the prepared loaf tin and scatter the mixed seeds over the top. Place in the oven and bake for around 70 minutes, or until you can stick a skewer or sharp knife into the loaf and it comes out clean.

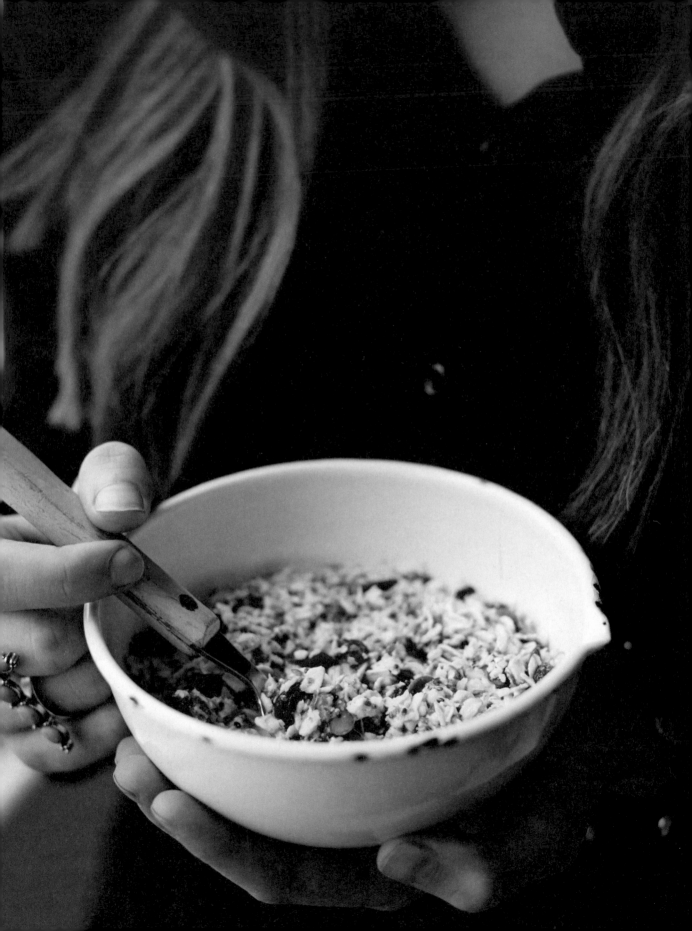

Flax and goji berry muesli

MAKES 8 SERVINGS

200g (2 cups) (gluten-free)
  rolled oats
35g (¼ cup) ground flaxseeds
90g (½ cup) Medjool dates,
  pitted and chopped
55g (½ cup) dried goji berries
140g (1 cup) pumpkin seeds
40g (½ cup) desiccated
  coconut
40g (¼ cup) chia seeds

Muesli is supposed to be a healthier type of breakfast cereal, but personally I think some varieties just taste like cardboard! Absolutely no flavour and, what's more, not all that nutritious. This muesli is quite the reverse – super-tasty and bursting with goodness. It's something I always have sitting in my pantry to turn to on those mornings where muesli and piping hot almond milk is called for – which happens all too often.

Simply add all the ingredients to a mixing bowl, mix together and pour into an airtight container. It will keep like this for up to 4 weeks.

SWITCH IT UP

These ingredients are also delicious made into a granola. Mix the ingredients together as above, excluding the goji berries. Add 60ml (¼ cup) pure maple syrup, toss together and bake in the oven for 25 minutes at 180°C/160°C fan/ gas 3. Remove from the oven and mix in the goji berries before allowing to cool and storing in an airtight container.

Golden granola and coconut cream parfait

SERVES 4–6

Granola
120g (1 cup) raw cashews
115g (1 cup) pecans
2 tablespoons chia seeds
25g (½ cup) coconut flakes
70g (½ cup) sultanas or
  raisins
200g (2 cups) (gluten-free)
  rolled oats
2 tablespoons raw cacao
  (or cocoa) powder
2 generous tablespoons
  coconut oil
60ml (¼ cup) pure
  maple syrup
1 teaspoon pure vanilla
  extract
2 teaspoons ground
  cinnamon

Whipped coconut cream
2 x 400ml tins of full-fat
  coconut milk
60ml (¼ cup) pure maple
  syrup

Parfait
120g (1 cup) raspberries,
  crushed

This granola parfait is honestly one of my favourite breakfasts. It is so incredibly delicious, and tastes so naughty, when in fact it's made with nothing but good-for-you ingredients. While, yes, there is a little preparing to do, the results are amazing and keep you going for ever! (See photo on page 1).

The day before you plan to make the granola parfait, empty the tins of coconut milk for the coconut cream into an airtight plastic container and place in the freezer for a couple of hours. Remove the container and scoop out the solidified/frozen cream (which will have separated from any watery liquid) into a bowl. When it has defrosted, transfer to a blender, add the maple syrup and blend for 3 minutes, then pour into a jar and chill in the fridge overnight before using.

When you are ready to make the granola parfait, preheat the oven to 180°C/160°C fan/gas 4 and line a baking tray with baking parchment.

To make the granola, start by chopping your cashews and pecans into smaller chunks. (To save time, you can quickly pulse them in a food processor.) Mix in a bowl with the chia seeds, coconut flakes, sultanas or raisins, oats and cacao (or cocoa) powder.

In a saucepan, combine the coconut oil, maple syrup, vanilla extract and cinnamon over a medium-low heat. Heat until the coconut oil is melted, then pour into the dry ingredients and mix until everything is well coated. Tip the mixture into the prepared baking tray, spreading it out in an even layer, and place in the oven to cook for around half an hour or until golden brown.

To assemble the parfait, place half the crushed raspberries in a serving bowl, add the granola in an even layer, followed by the remaining raspberries, and top with the coconut cream (having given this a quick stir first).

SWITCH IT UP

As long as you keep the oat and coconut cream quantities the same for the granola, you can change any of the other ingredients. Use any nuts, seeds or dried fruit you like. Blueberries, sliced banana, strawberries or pomegranate seeds could all be used instead of the raspberries. And if you're not keen on coconut, try this recipe with my mango-cashew cream (see page 50) instead. It's perfect for summer and so vibrant-tasting. However you ring the changes, this dish always tastes delicious and never fails to please.

Mini berry breakfast crumble

SERVES 1

125g (1 cup) blueberries
60g (½ cup) raspberries
60ml (¼ cup) dairy-free milk
    of your choice (to make
    your own, see pages 74–75)
1 tablespoon sultanas
2 teaspoons ground
    cinnamon
1 teaspoon pure vanilla
    extract

Crumble topping
50g (½ cup) (gluten-free)
    rolled oats
1 tablespoon pure
    maple syrup
1 tablespoon pumpkin seeds

Crumble for breakfast? Surely not! This mini breakfast crumble is, hands down, one of my favourite breakfasts. I'm not quite sure why, as this book is full of incredible recipes, but I particularly love the flavours here, their clear-cut simplicity, and the fact that it's crumble ... And who doesn't love crumble!

Preheat the oven to 190°C/170°C fan/gas 5. Place the blueberries and raspberries in a saucepan with the milk over a medium-high heat. When the blueberries have softened but just before they begin to pop, add the sultanas, cinnamon and vanilla extract and stir to combine. Remove from the heat and transfer the gooey mixture into the bottom of a small dish (such as a ramekin).

Next mix together all the ingredients for the crumble topping and place this in a layer on top of the blueberry mixture in the ramekin. Pop in the oven and cook for 10–15 minutes, or until the top begins to brown.

SWITCH IT UP

Blueberries and raspberries make this mini breakfast crumble berry-licious, but if you're a bigger fan of apple crumble, you can use one apple and a handful of berries for a more classic combo.

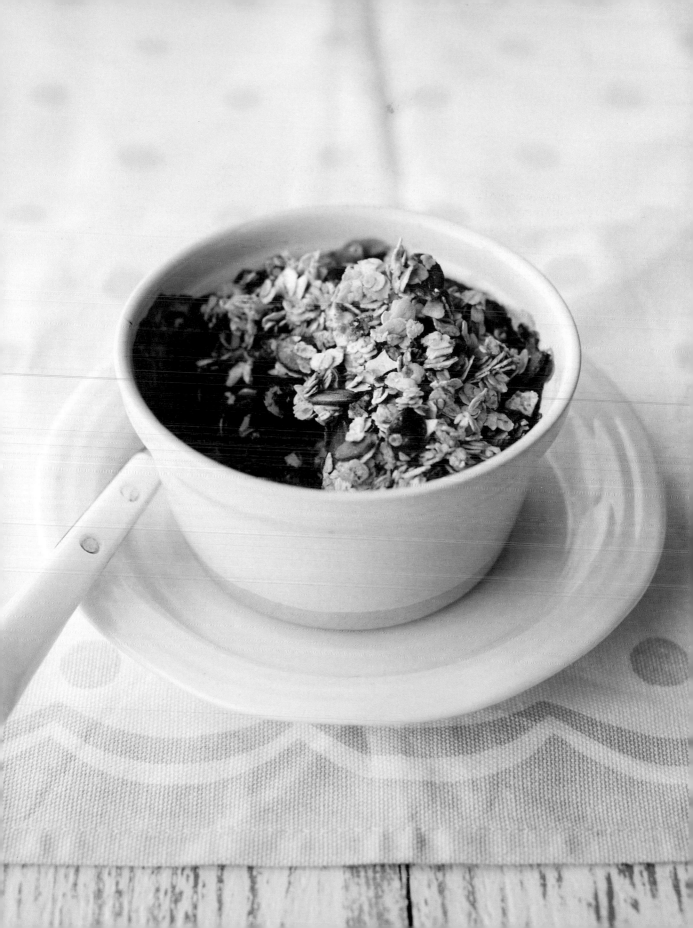

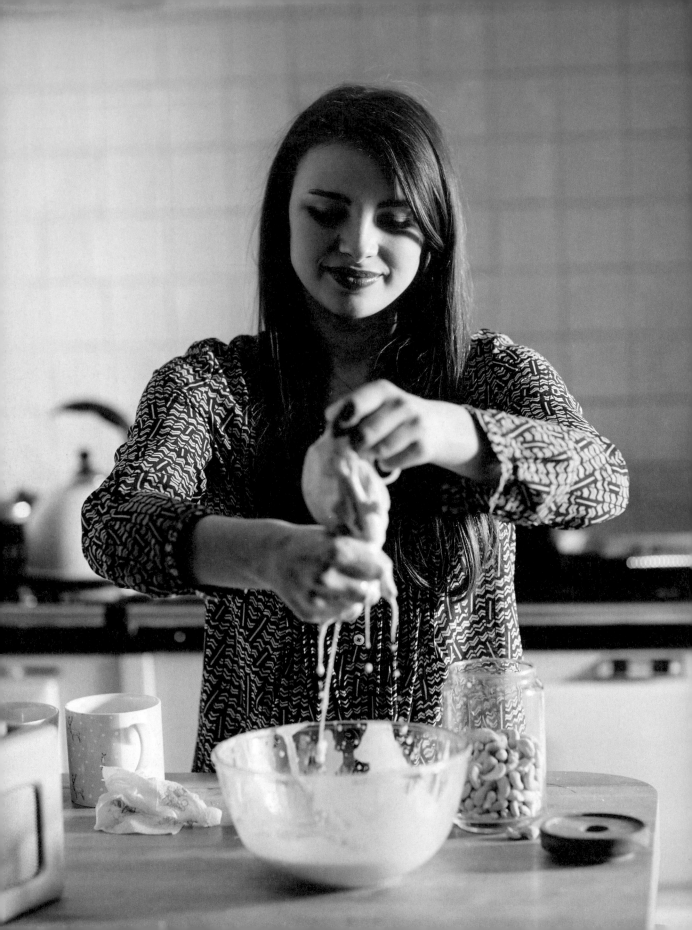

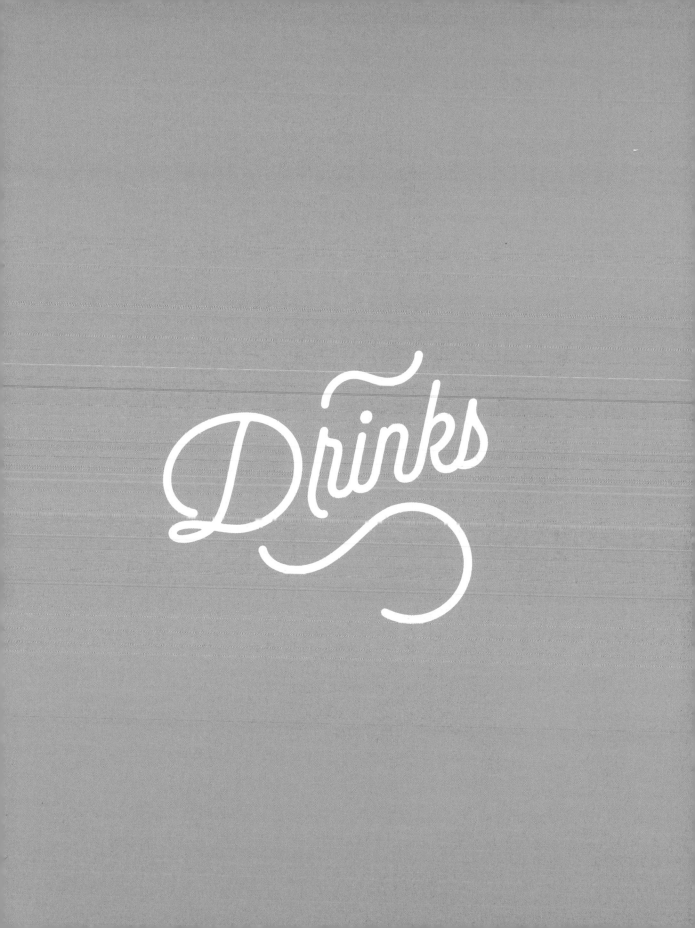

When you begin to eat unrefined, unprocessed foods, kick-starting a much healthier diet, it's easy to forget that what you drink is just as important.

Having a Diet Coke alongside a superfood salad doesn't cancel out the E-numbers and additives in the Coke (even if we wish it did). This chapter is all about drinks that taste as good as the fantastic ingredients they're made with and I'm just so excited to be sharing the recipes with you.

They are all so easy to prepare, requiring only a little more effort than running to the store to buy a multi-pack of fizzy drinks. They make great breakfasts, wonderful snacks or a soothing, warming treat before bed. Perfect for any time of day, they are also a wonderful way to begin experimenting with new flavours.

For ease of reference, I've divided this chapter into different sections, starting with 'How to Make Dairy-Free Milk' (see page 74), as it forms the basis of so many drinks and can be made in lots of different flavours – chocolate being my favourite!

Then it's 'Hot Drinks' (see page 76), which are perfect for two things, firstly to replace that morning cup of coffee and secondly to provide that bit of comfort at the end of a long day. While, yes, caffeine does wake us up first thing in the morning, the reliance we have on it is due entirely to habit. The real draw of coffee, other than that electric burst of energy, is the warmth and comfort it provides, the boost it gives you to tackle the day ahead. It's addictive, and not just for your body, but for your mind. The hot drinks in this section will help to wean you from that addiction, I promise. The first step is to buy a 'to go' cup, so you can make your drink at home and take it on the commute with you. The second step is to be open-minded – give it a week or two and, slowly but surely, you will start to love the flavour of your new drink even if you initially loathed it.

After 'Hot Drinks' it's 'Smoothies and Juices' (see pages 78–82), further subdivided into 'Energise' and 'Cleanse' (see pages 78–81), to highlight the benefits of those particular drinks. At the end of most of the recipes, I've given a few twists suggesting alternative ingredients, so you can see how easy it is to experiment using whatever you have in the fridge or can easily buy from your local supermarket.

Opposite, from left to right: Raw chocolate milkshake, Anti-inflammatory gingerbread smoothie, Almond butter 'caramel' protein smoothie, Energising berry-cashew smoothie.

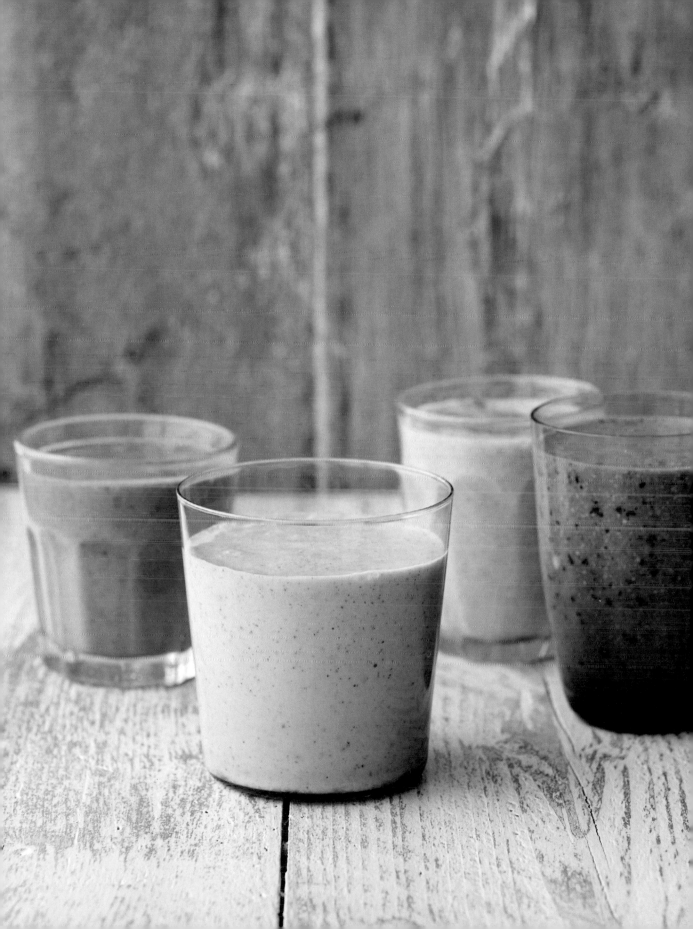

HOW TO MAKE

Dairy-Free Milk

A good dairy-free milk is essential, whether it's for a bowl of Golden Granola (see page 66) or just a drizzle in a cup of rooibos tea – my fridge is never without a jugful. There are lots of different bases you can choose from for your homemade milk – almonds, cashews, brazil nuts, desiccated coconut, brown rice or oats – and I've suggested four delicious flavourings too. Once you've got the hang of making it, you can experiment with other base ingredients or flavourings to ring the changes. This basic recipe makes 1 litre (4¼ cups) milk, though in my house it goes so quickly I always end up doubling the recipe!

MAKES ABOUT 1 LITRE (4¼ CUPS)
DAIRY-FREE MILK

BASE
Choose one of the following:
130g (1 cup) whole almonds
120g (1 cup) raw cashews
125g (1 cup) brazil nuts
200g (2 cups) (gluten-free) rolled oats
200g (2½ cups) desiccated coconut
190g (1 cup) brown rice

LIQUID
1 litre (4¼ cups) water

SWEETENER (OPTIONAL)
Choose one of the following:

2–4 Medjool dates, pitted and chopped
    (my favourite!)
1–3 tablespoons raw honey,
    agave or pure maple syrup

FLAVOURING (OPTIONAL)
Choose one of the following:
Vanilla
1 teaspoon pure vanilla extract
Chocolate
2 tablespoons raw cacao (or cocoa) powder
Strawberry
70g (⅔ cup) strawberries, hulled
Banana
1 medium-sized banana, peeled and sliced

METHOD

1 If using nuts or oats as your base, start by soaking these in water for at least 2 hours or preferably overnight, then drain. If using desiccated coconut, no preparation is needed.

2 If using brown rice, you'll need to cook it first. Add to a saucepan with 475ml (2 cups) water and a pinch of salt and bring to the boil. Reduce the heat and simmer for 40–50 minutes until the water is fully absorbed (you can add more during cooking, if needed) and the rice is light and fluffy.

3 Add your chosen base to a high-powered blender or a food processor with the water, sweetener (if using) and flavouring, if making flavoured milk. Blend until smooth – around 3 minutes – and then strain through a muslin cloth or a nut-milk bag. Pour into an airtight container and store in the fridge for up to 4 days for nut milk and 6 days for oat or rice milk.

Superfood hot chocolate

I've loved this hot chocolate for years and can't remember a week I haven't had it at least once.

SERVES 1

240ml (1 cup) almond milk (or oat
    or brown rice milk – to make your
    own, see pages 74–75)
1 tablespoon raw cacao (or cocoa) powder
1 tablespoon pure maple syrup
1 teaspoon almond butter
1 teaspoon bee pollen (optional)

In a saucepan, combine the almond milk, cacao (or cocoa) powder, maple syrup and almond butter. Place the pan on a medium heat and, just before the milk starts to bubble, pour into your favourite mug and sprinkle over the bee pollen.

Turmeric and cinnamon mylk

Turmeric is one of my favourite spices.

SERVES 1

240ml (1 cup) almond milk
½–1 tablespoon raw honey,
    agave or pure maple syrup
½ teaspoon turmeric
½ teaspoon ground cinnamon

Add all the ingredients to a saucepan and place on a medium heat. Heat through, stirring constantly, until the milk starts to bubble, then pour into a glass and enjoy!

Matcha latte

I was introduced to a matcha latte last year and absolutely loathed it. But as I was in the process of weaning myself off coffee, I needed an alternative and so I persevered. By making my own matcha latte I got the flavour just right. With a little sweetener and the right dairy-free milk, it's yummy.

SERVES 1

½ teaspoon matcha powder
240ml (1 cup) dairy-free milk of your choice
    (to make your own, see pages 74–75)
½ teaspoon pure vanilla extract (optional)
½ tablespoon raw honey, agave
    or pure maple syrup

Place the matcha powder in a cup and whisk with 2–3cm of hot water until smooth. Add the milk to a saucepan with the vanilla extract (if using) and raw honey or agave/maple syrup and heat through, stirring as you go. Bring just to the boil, then remove from the heat.

Slowly pour into the cup with the matcha paste, stirring all the time so no lumps form, and adding a little more honey, to sweeten, if needed.

Opposite, clockwise from top: Matcha latte , Turmeric and cinnamon mylk, Superfood hot chocolate.

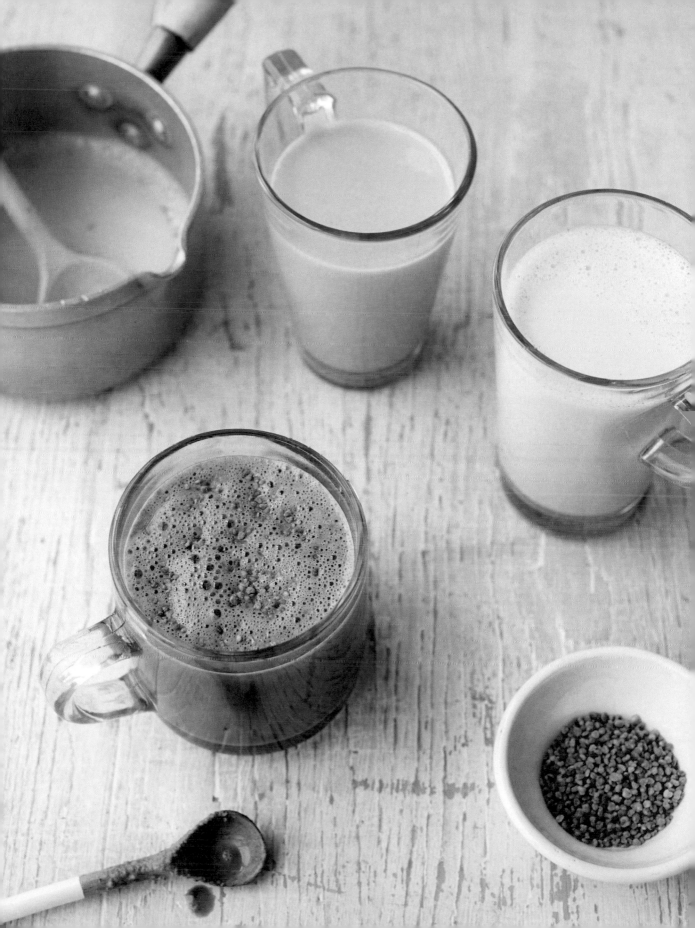

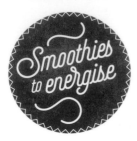

Smoothies to energise

Raw chocolate milkshake

This smoothie is absolutely divine, and so rich and velvety that it's hard to believe it's so good for you! The chocolate flavour hides the fact that it's also chock-full of healthy fats and amino acids, supplying you with an incredible source of energy. I love it for a (not so) naughty breakfast.

SERVES 1

1 banana, peeled, sliced and frozen
    (or you can use a fresh banana)
½ avocado, peeled and stoned
3 Medjool dates, pitted and chopped
1 tablespoon raw cacao (or cocoa) powder
1 tablespoon almond butter (optional)
350ml (1½ cups) almond, rice or oat milk
    (to make your own, see pages 74–75)

Place all the ingredients in a high-powered blender or food processor and blend until smooth.

SWITCH IT UP

You can omit the avocado for a thinner smoothie, or substitute with another half a banana. Completely up to you!

Energising berry-cashew smoothie

Berry smoothies are a great way to up your antioxidants in the morning, as well as boosting your immune system and providing lots of long-lasting energy. They can also be frozen in batches, which is both cost effective and means you don't have to rush out for ingredients every time you fancy making one.

1 banana, peeled, sliced and frozen
    (or you can use a fresh banana)
30g (¼ cup) raw cashews, soaked in water for
    at least 2 hours or overnight, then drained
240ml (1 cup) almond milk (or any diary-
    free milk you like – to make your own,
    see pages 74–75)
60g (½ cup) blueberries
60g (½ cup) raspberries
2 teaspoons acai berry powder (optional)
1 tablespoon chia seeds (optional)

Place all the ingredients in a high-powered blender or a food processor and blend until smooth.

SWITCH IT UP

Although blueberries and raspberries are perfect in this smoothie, don't feel restricted to using only them. You can substitute with any other berries you like, keeping to a similar quantity of at least 120g (¾–1 cup). Why not try strawberries, blackberries or even pomegranate seeds? While cashews are my favourite, you can also use Brazil nuts or, if you're allergic to nuts, sunflower seeds!

Almond butter 'caramel' protein smoothie

This smoothie has been a favourite of mine for a really long time. Not only does it taste incredible, it's also a great way to pile in the protein pre- or post-workout.

SERVES 1–2

1 large banana, peeled, sliced and frozen
1 heaped teaspoon brown rice protein powder
350ml (1½ cups) almond milk
2 Medjool dates, pitted and chopped
1 tablespoon almond butter

Optional
¼ teaspoon pure vanilla extract
Pinch of ground cinnamon

Place all the ingredients in a high-powered blender or a food processor and blend until smooth.

SWITCH IT UP

If you're not an almond butter fan, try using peanut or cashew butter instead. (To make your own nut butter, see page 58.)

TIP

The flavour of protein powder varies according to the brand and hence will affect the taste of your smoothie, so it's important to make sure you like the type you've chosen. The Sunwarrior and Pulsin brands are favourites of mine.

Anti-inflammatory gingerbread smoothie

I'm a big fan of anything sweet and gingery, and this smoothie is both of these. The combination is just so delicious and tastes and smells like homemade gingerbread – a smell I remember vividly growing up! This recipe will not only energise you, but has a wonderfully alkalising effect, reducing acidity and restoring the pH balance, as well as calming down any inflammation in the body.

SERVES 1

1 banana, peeled
25g (¼ cup) (gluten-free) rolled oats
1 teaspoon peeled and finely chopped
   fresh root ginger
1 teaspoon ground cinnamon
180ml (¾ cup) almond milk
1 tablespoon almond butter (optional)

Add all the ingredients to your blender and blend!

(All recipes photographed on page 73)

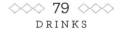

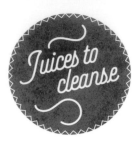
Juices to cleanse

Beetroot, carrot, pineapple and ginger juice

Not only is this a super-powerful cleansing tonic, it's super-tasty too. Pineapple, carrot, lemon, beetroot and ginger are all incredible anti-inflammatories in their own right, so together they are a force to be reckoned with! (See photo on page 83).

SERVES 1

2 carrots
1 beetroot
400g (2 cups) peeled and
    chopped fresh pineapple
1 thumbnail-sized knob of fresh
    root ginger, peeled
Juice of ½ lemon

Wash the carrots and beetroot thoroughly, or peel them, then put through your juicer with the pineapple and ginger before mixing with the lemon juice.

SWITCH IT UP

You can substitute the carrots for another beta-carotene-rich vegetable, such as sweet potato.

The perfect green juice

I've tried a lot of green juices and this one remains my favourite. It's the perfect balance, packed with astringent greens yet sweet and refreshing, and certainly not a challenge to drink! I tend to make two batches and keep the other in an airtight container for the next morning. (See photo on page 83).

SERVES 2

2 eating apples
1 cucumber
2 handfuls of broccoli florets
4 stalks of celery
2 handfuls of spinach
2 handfuls of chopped kale
Juice of ½ lemon
1 thumbnail-sized knob of fresh
    root ginger, peeled

Wash the apples and vegetables thoroughly, then put through a juicer with the remaining ingredients – and enjoy!

SWITCH IT UP

Try replacing the apple with a pear or 400g (2 cups) of peeled and chopped fresh pineapple. You can also replace the kale and spinach with the same quantity of any seasonal leafy greens. And, instead of the lemon, why not try a lime! (You'd need the juice of 1 lime for the ½ lemon here.)

Carrot, orange and turmeric tonic

This juice is exactly as the recipe title indicates: a cleansing tonic that doesn't just taste delicious but is so wonderful for you. Packed with vitamin C and beta-carotene, it's my 'go to' when I start to get that fluey feeling. (See photo on page 83).

SERVES 1–2

3 medium-sized carrots
2 medium-sized oranges, peeled
1 thumbnail-sized knob of fresh
    root ginger, peeled
½ teaspoon turmeric

Wash or peel the carrots and put through a juicer with the oranges and ginger. Place the turmeric in a glass with a drop of water and mix into a paste, then slowly pour in the juice, stirring as you go. This ensures that the juice remains lovely and smooth, and not lumpy, as it would if you added the turmeric to the juice after pouring it out.

SWITCH IT UP

Why not try sweet potatoes or beetroot instead of the carrots, or swap the oranges for apples or pears?

Glowing green smoothie

I always feel so good after starting the day with a green smoothie, It sets me up for the day ahead and gives me the most amazing sense of alertness. The balance here is just right, with enough protein to sustain you while also balancing those blood-sugar levels. (See photo on page 224).

SERVES 1

1 banana, peeled
1–2 Medjool dates, pitted and chopped
40g (⅓ cup) raw cashews, soaked in
    water for at least 2 hours or overnight,
    then drained
1 handful each of spinach and
    chopped kale (stems removed)
400ml (1¾ cups) coconut water

Add all the ingredients to a high-powered blender or a food processor and blend.

SWITCH IT UP

Why not try half an avocado instead of the banana? To replace the cashews, you could use brazil nuts, or sunflower seeds if you have a nut allergy.

Berry burst smoothie

This smoothie is my summer 'go to'; it's just so refreshing. Easy to make in big batches for your family and friends, it's a real crowd pleaser too. (See photo on page 224).

SERVES 2

1 banana, peeled, sliced and frozen
60g (½ cup) blueberries
60g (⅓ cup) pomegranate seeds
1 tablespoon ground flaxseeds
2 teaspoons acai berry powder (optional)
80ml (⅓ cup) dairy-free milk of your choice
    (to make your own, see pages 74–75)

Add everything to a high-powered blender or a food processor and blend.

SWITCH IT UP

In this recipe, you can use 75–90g (½–¾ cup) of any berries of your choice – don't feel limited to only blueberries and pomegranate seeds. Why not try raspberries, strawberries or blackberries? To replace the flaxseeds, you could try using chia seeds, 1 tablespoon of nut butter, or a handful of nuts or seeds.

Sunshine smoothie

This is the essence of sunshine – the colour is so vibrant and the taste is like that of no other smoothie. There are only three ingredients, too, with a few optional extras. It's the perfect summer smoothie.

SERVES 1

1 mango, peeled, stoned and cubed
1 banana, peeled, sliced and frozen
Juice of 1 orange

Extras (optional)
1 tablespoon chia seeds
2 tablespoons (gluten-free) rolled oats
1 tablespoon cashew butter

Add everything to a high-powered blender or a food processor and blend.

Opposite, from left to right: Sunshine smoothie, The perfect green juice, Beetroot, carrot, pineapple and ginger juice, Carrot, orange and turmeric tonic.

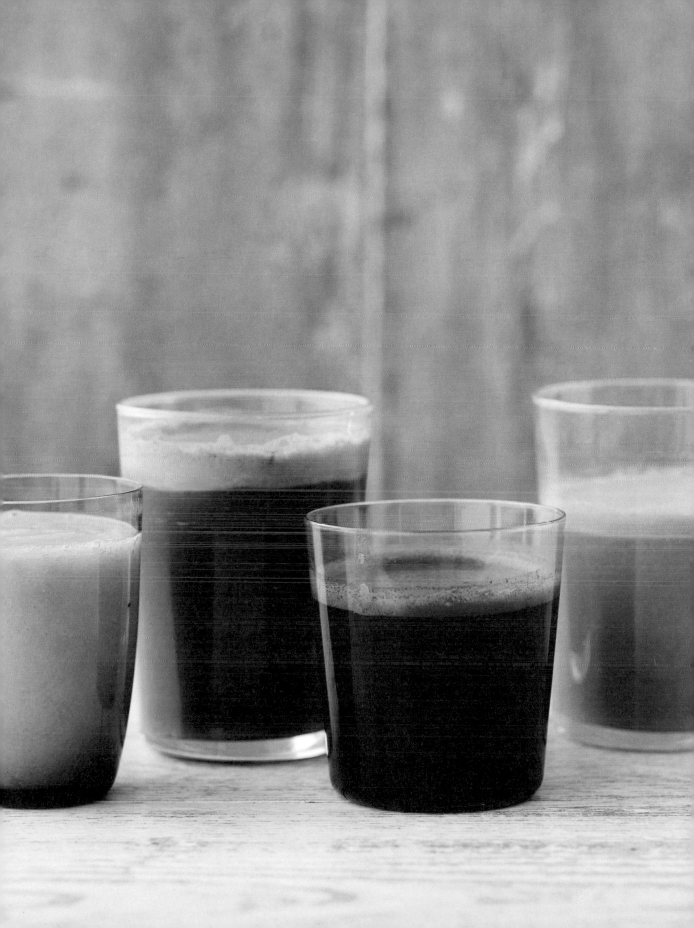

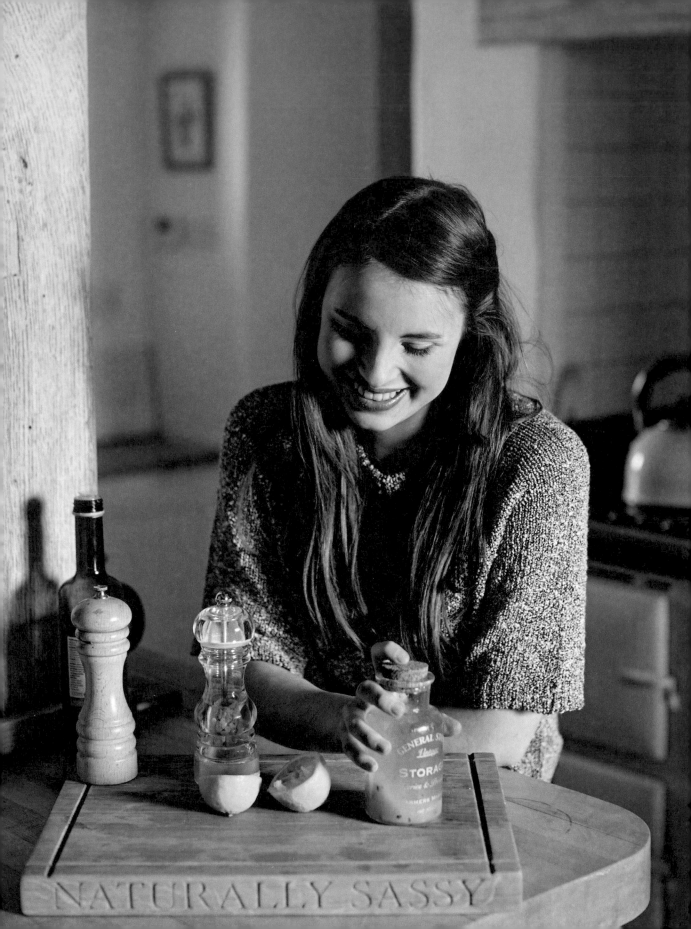

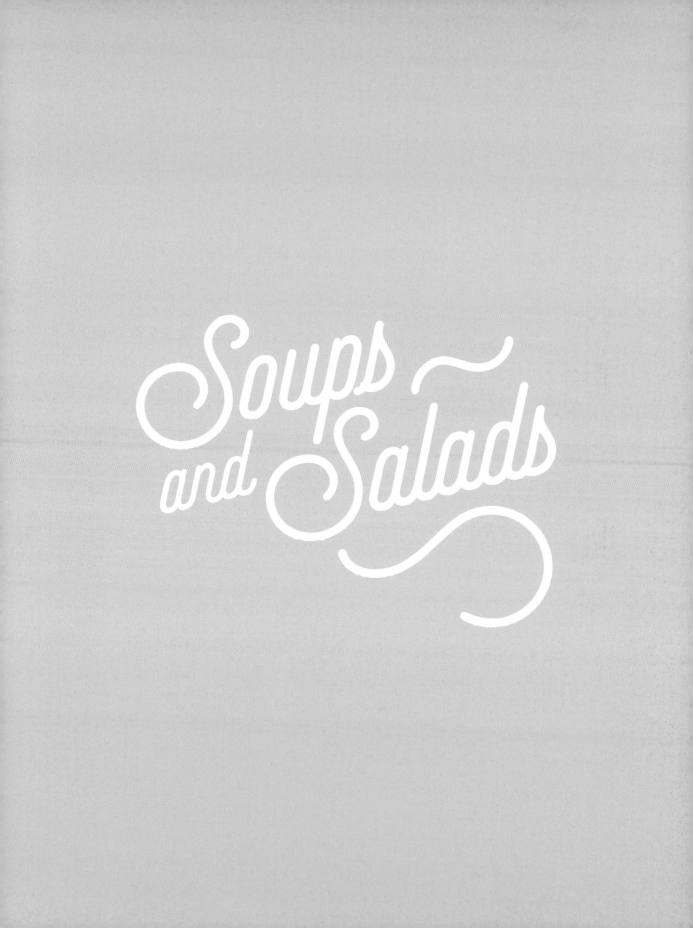

Soups ~ and Salads

Lunch can be a hard meal to get right when it comes to eating well.

When I changed my diet, I found this middle meal of the day really hard to get right. As a dancer, I was always dashing from class to class, with no time to hunt out a healthy salad in the parade of fast-food shops by the studio. So I decided it would be better to bring food with me. I was at that point pretty unadventurous and ended up eating iceberg lettuce and sweet potatoes with sunflower seeds for a good month or so. It was tiresome. Then one day I opened my lunch box and just reeled at the sight of iceberg lettuce yet again; I knew something had to change if I was going to continue bringing food with me for a healthy lunch. That weekend, I played around with different ideas for the week ahead, experimenting with minimal ingredients. I did this each Sunday, until I started to enjoy the hour or so I spent gathering everything together.

In the 'Sunday Prep' section at the end of this chapter (see pages 109–111), I've shown you how to prepare a range of items to mix and match for the week ahead so that you too can get to love your lunch box and eat well every day. There are lots of small components that make up a really great packed lunch. With practice, you can make them all in under an hour at the weekend. Store them in the fridge, so you can pick and mix all the different components – making something different each day.

If you're eating lunch at home, or if you're looking for a light supper or a salad to eat as part of a larger meal, you may prefer to make one of my more complex salads from the first section in this chapter. From spiralised beetroot or marinated pesto-courgette ribbons to lemon-infused wild rice (see pages 93, 97 and 104), they are full of gloriously contrasting flavours and textures. While they can be made fresh to eat the same day, they can also be prepared well in advance. You could make one 'to go' the following day, for instance, or as part of your Sunday prep, swapping it for one of the salads in that section and mixing and matching with the other salads there. I make two big salads and store them in plastic containers. Then I add a big spoonful of each to my lunch box.

For cooler days, there are soups. So satisfying and full of flavour, they are a great way to pack in tons of healthy veg. I love my soups thick and creamy, with lots of sweet root vegetables – like the Beetroot and butternut soup or the Sweet potato and leek soup (see pages 88 and 89). They're a great way to refuel for a midday meal at home, but also a fantastic option to take with you as a packed lunch. As part of my Sunday prep, I'll sometimes make a big batch of soup and store it in the fridge. Then just before I leave for work, I'll heat up a single portion and put it in a flask, so it's piping hot for a wonderfully nourishing lunch on the go.

Spicy red pepper soup

SERVES 4

1 large butternut squash, peeled, deseeded and cut into small cubes

2 large or 3 small sweet potatoes, peeled and cut into small cubes

2 red peppers, deseeded and sliced

2 tablespoons olive oil

Leaves from 1 sprig of rosemary or thyme

350ml (1½ cups) water

120ml (½ cup) full-fat coconut milk

2 teaspoons apple cider vinegar (optional)

Juice of 1 lime

1 teaspoon deseeded and finely chopped red chilli (or to taste)

Salt and pepper

TIP

If you're using a standard blender for blending the cooked vegetables, it's best to whizz them in 2–3 small batches.

Eaten raw, red peppers are not my favourite vegetable, but roasted they are incredibly tasty and add an amazing flavour to this soup. Instead of the cream or full-fat milk that's commonly added to soup, I use coconut milk to give that extra creaminess. The effect is magical, taking this soup from merely delicious to extraordinary. (See photo on page 91).

◇◇◇◇◇◇◇◇◇◇◇◇◇◇◇◇◇◇◇◇◇◇◇◇◇◇◇◇◇◇◇◇◇◇

Preheat the oven to 190°C/170°C fan/gas 5. Place the squash, sweet potatoes and peppers in a roasting tin, spread out in an even layer. Add the olive oil, a pinch of salt and a sprinkling of rosemary or thyme leaves, then place in the oven to roast for around 30 minutes, until soft.

Once cooked, place the squash, sweet potatoes and peppers in a high-powered blender or food processor with the remaining ingredients, then blend until smooth.

Pour into a saucepan and heat until piping hot, adding more water and coconut milk if you prefer a slightly thinner soup. Season to taste with salt and pepper and serve immediately.

Beetroot and butternut soup

SERVES 4–6

2 large beetroots, peeled
    and chopped
1 medium-sized butternut
    squash, peeled, deseeded
    and chopped
60ml (¼ cup) full-fat
    coconut milk
1 thumbnail-sized knob
    of fresh root ginger,
    peeled and grated
700ml (3 cups) vegetable
    stock (made with a stock
    cube or bouillon powder)
Salt and pepper

Not only is this soup a beautiful vibrant colour, it's packed with beety flavour, and combined with the creaminess the of the butternut squash, it makes a really delicious, hearty bowl of soup. (See photo on page 91).

◇◇◇◇◇◇◇◇◇◇◇◇◇◇◇◇◇◇◇◇◇◇◇◇◇◇◇◇◇◇◇◇◇◇◇

Steam the chopped beetroot and butternut squash over a high heat for 25 minutes until tender. Place in a blender with the coconut milk, ginger and vegetable stock and blend until smooth, seasoning with salt and pepper to taste. Pour into a saucepan and heat through until piping hot, then divide between bowls to serve.

SWITCH IT UP

Peeling, deseeding and chopping up a squash can sometimes be a bit of a faff. To save time, you can use ready-cubed squash or even switch it for 2 large sweet potatoes.

Sweet potato and leek soup with chilli-roasted seeds

SERVES 4–6

4 medium-sized sweet
   potatoes, peeled and
   cut into small cubes
4 tablespoons olive oil
Pinch of salt
2 large leeks, chopped
1 thumbnail-sized knob
   of fresh root ginger,
   peeled and grated
60ml (¼ cup) full-fat
   coconut milk
1.5 litres (6 cups) vegetable
   stock (made with a stock
   cube or bouillon powder)

Chilli-roasted seeds
35g (¼ cup) mixed seeds
   (such as sesame, pumpkin
   and sunflower)
½ tablespoon tamari
Pinch of chilli flakes

TIP

If you're making this soup
a few days in advance 'to go'
then don't add the roasted
seeds but take them with you
to add to your soup when
you pour it out of the flask.

Soups are so underrated, it's easy to forget how
amazing they can taste. Because the ingredients
are cooked and puréed, they are really easy to
digest, too. I like my soups thick, creamy, piping
hot and packed with flavour. Vegetables like squash
and sweet potato give real body to a soup, which
I love, as well as a wonderful sweetness. (See
photo on page 91).

Preheat the oven to 190°C/170°C fan/gas 5. Spread
the sweet potatoes out in a roasting tin, add the olive
oil and a pinch of salt and roast in the oven for about
30 minutes or until soft.

While the sweet potatoes are roasting, prepare the
seeds. Mix the seeds, tamari and chilli flakes together,
scatter into a small roasting tin or baking tray and
place in the oven to roast for around 3 minutes,
shaking the tin once or twice to ensure they don't
burn. Remove from the oven and set aside to cool.

Pour the remaining olive oil into a pan and fry the
leeks over a medium high heat for 3–4 minutes until
softened and slightly caramelised, then remove from
the heat and set aside.

When the sweet potatoes are cooked, add to a
blender with the leeks, ginger, coconut milk and
vegetable stock and whizz until smooth. Pour into
a saucepan and heat through until piping hot, then
divide between bowls and scatter over the mixed
seeds to serve.

Following page, from top left: Spicy
red pepper soup, Beetroot and butternut
soup, Avocado gazpacho, Sweet potato
and leek soup with chilli-roasted seeds.

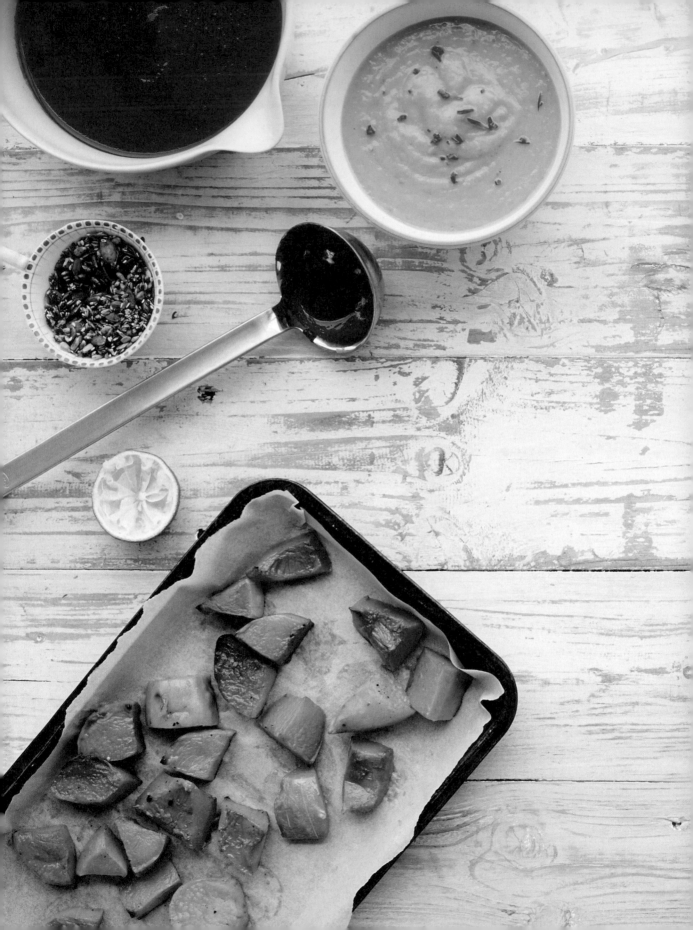

Avocado gazpacho

SERVES 2-4

1 cucumber, peeled
   and chopped
1 avocado, peeled and stoned
3 tablespoons fresh
   lemon juice
1 handful of fresh coriander
1 jalapeño pepper, deseeded
120ml (½ cup) full-fat
   coconut milk
240ml (1 cup) ice-cold water
1½ teaspoons salt

Incredibly fresh and packed full of nutrients, this is the perfect summer soup. The combination of avocado and coconut cream makes it very creamy and filling – ideal for a slightly lighter meal that will nonetheless keep you satisfied through the afternoon.

Add everything to your blender and blend!

Kale salad with maple roasted walnuts, cranberries and citrus-sesame dressing

2 medium-sized sweet
    potatoes, peeled and
    cut into small cubes
1–2 tablespoons olive oil
1 teaspoon ground cinnamon
Generous pinch of salt
1 x 180g bag of kale
1 large avocado
25g (¼ cup) dried
    cranberries

Tahini dressing
2 tablespoons tahini
2 tablespoons extra-virgin
    olive oil
Juice of ½ lemon
Juice of ½ large orange
½ tablespoon tamari
    (or to taste)
1 tablespoon nutritional yeast
    (optional)

Maple roasted walnuts
50g (½ cup) walnut halves
1 generous tablespoon pure
    maple syrup
1 generous tablespoon
    olive oil

TIP
If you're making this salad
a few days in advance 'to
go' then omit the kale and
avocado, adding them to
your lunch box, along with
a portion of the salad, the
night before and storing
in the fridge.

Raw kale in a salad may not sound very appetising, but with a little bit of magic it becomes truly delicious. The secret is a thick, creamy, tastebud-tingling dressing and a massage ... Not for you – for the kale! However bizarre this may sound, massaging the kale allows the dressing to coat the leaves, making the kale soft and easy to eat. (See photo on page 94).

Preheat the oven to 190°C/170°C fan/gas 5. Spread the sweet potatoes out in a roasting tin, drizzle with olive oil, sprinkle with the cinnamon and salt, and place in the oven to bake for around 30 minutes or until soft.

Meanwhile, wash the kale, drying the leaves well and removing any hard stems. Mix all ingredients for the dressing in a large bowl, add the kale and massage the dressing into the leaves for around 3 minutes, until they soften/wilt.

Place the walnuts in a bowl with the maple syrup and olive oil, mix well and add to the sweet potatoes in the roasting tin 2–3 minutes before removing from the oven.

Peel and stone the avocado and cut into cubes, then add to the salad with the cranberries and the roasted sweet potatoes (reserving the toasted walnuts). Toss well, and divide between plates, sprinkling with the walnuts.

SWITCH IT UP
You can swap the sweet potato for butternut squash, and the cranberries for pomegranate seeds.

Beetroot, lentil and pine nut salad with a balsamic lemon vinaigrette

SERVES 2

100g (½ cup) dried
   beluga lentils
30g (¼ cup) pine nuts
5 beetroots, peeled
50g (⅓ cup) raisins

Dressing
Juice of 1 lemon
2 tablespoons balsamic
   vinegar
1 teaspoon agave or
   pure maple syrup
Pinch of salt

TIP

If you're pushed for time, you can use ready-cooked beluga lentils, available from the supermarket.

This salad is made with my trusty friend, a spiraliser, a wonderful device that can turn vegetables into spaghetti and make any meal feel that little bit more creative. It's an affordable piece of equipment, and one of my best investments. If you don't have have a spiraliser, that's absolutely fine – simply grate the beetroot, or peel it into strips. (See photo on page 95).

◇◇◇◇◇◇◇◇◇◇◇◇◇◇◇◇◇◇◇◇◇◇◇◇◇◇◇◇

Start by putting the lentils on to cook. Place in a saucepan, cover with water and bring to the boil, then lower the heat to a simmer and cook for 20–25 minutes until tender. When cooked, drain the lentils and rinse with cold water.

To prepare the pine nuts, either roast in a baking tray in the oven (preheated to 190°C/170°C fan/gas 5) for 5 minutes until golden brown, shaking once or twice to ensure they don't burn, or in a pan on the hob.

Meanwhile, prepare the beetroots by either putting them through a spiraliser, if you have one, grating them or using a vegetable peeler to peel them into fine strips.

Add the spiralised beetroot to a large bowl with the raisins, cooked lentils and toasted pine nuts. In a jug or separate small bowl, mix all ingredients for the dressing and then pour into the bowl with the salad, toss together well and plate up.

SWITCH IT UP

If you're not a beetroot lover, you can change it for the same quantity of carrots or courgettes.

Following page, clockwise from top left: Kale salad with maple roasted walnuts, cranberries and citrus-sesame dressing, Beetroot, lentil and pine nut salad with a balsamic lemon vinaigrette, Lemon quinoa tabbouleh with carrot, red pepper and avocado.

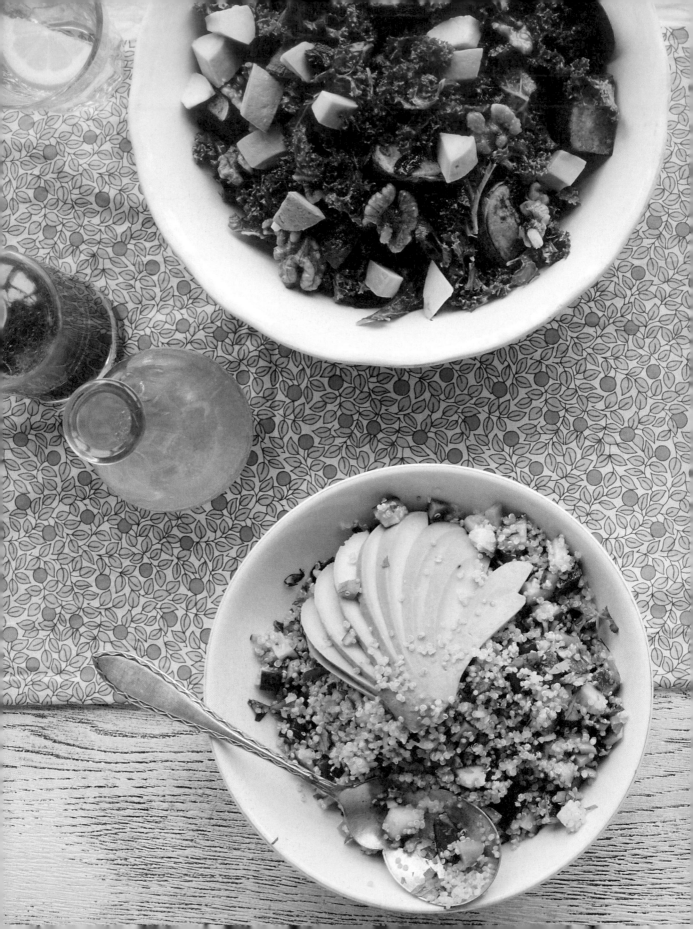

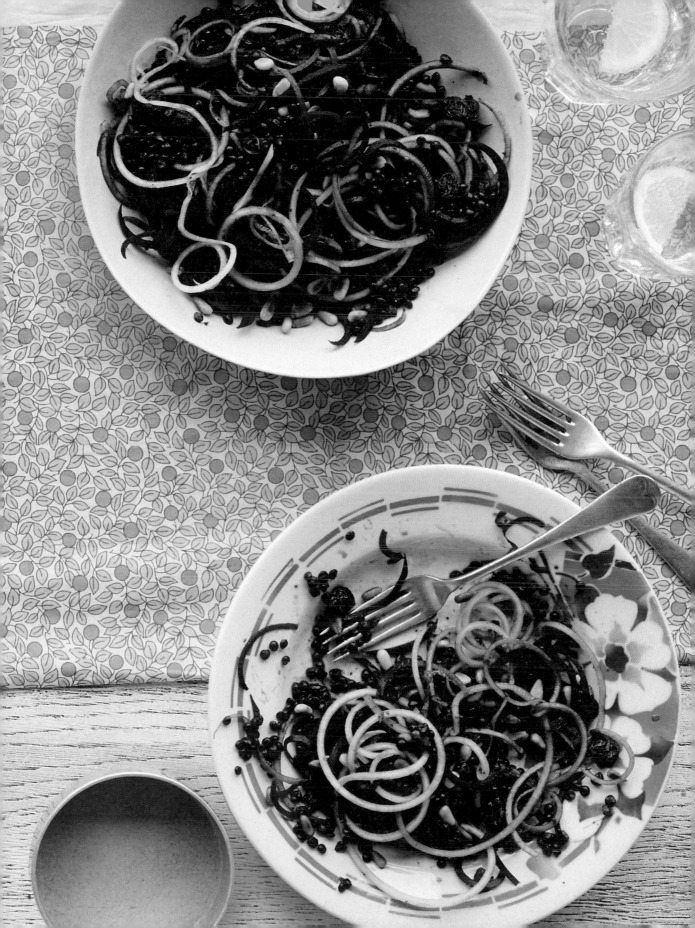

Lemon quinoa tabbouleh with carrot, red pepper and avocado

SERVES 4

Quinoa tabbouleh
170g (1 cup) quinoa
475ml (2 cups) boiling water
½ cucumber, finely diced
1 carrot, peeled and
    finely diced
1 red pepper, deseeded
    and diced
1 red onion, peeled and diced
3 tablespoons finely
    chopped coriander
Salt
1 avocado, peeled, stoned
    and sliced, to serve

Dressing
Juice of 1 lemon
1 tablespoon apple cider
    vinegar
2 tablespoons extra-virgin
    olive oil

TIP

If you're making this salad a few days in advance 'to go' then omit the avocado, adding it to your lunch box, along with a portion of the salad, the night before and storing in the fridge.

I love quinoa and this recipe is the perfect vehicle for showing off just how delicious it can be. Infused with lemon and apple cider vinegar, it offsets beautifully the earthier flavours of the vegetables. It keeps really well in the fridge, too, and as isn't an expensive dish to make as it's ideal for preparing as a larger batch, with enough left over for a speedy lunch on the go next day. (See photo on page 94).

Place the quinoa in a saucepan and add the water and a pinch of salt. Bring back up to the boil, then reduce the heat and simmer for 15–20 minutes or until light and fluffy, adding more water if needed. Remove from the heat and allow to cool.

Place in a large bowl with all the other ingredients for the tabbouleh, seasoning with salt to taste, and put to one side. Whisk together the ingredients for the dressing and pour over the quinoa mixture. Toss well together before plating up, topping with the avocado to serve.

SWITCH IT UP

If you're not too keen on quinoa, you can use millet or even brown rice. For the vegetables, feel free to use whatever raw, crunchy vegetables you like or have around.

Pesto-courgette ribbons, roasted squash and tamari pumpkin seeds

SERVES 2

1 medium-sized butternut
  squash, peeled, deseeded
  and cut into small cubes
1–2 tablespoons olive oil
Pinch of salt
4 courgettes

Pesto
90g (¾ cup) pine nuts
50g fresh basil
5 tablespoons extra-virgin
  olive oil
2 cloves of garlic, peeled
Generous pinch of salt
1 lemon

**Tamari-caramelised
pumpkin seeds**
50g (⅓ cup) pumpkin seeds
2 tablespoons tamari

TIP

If you're making this salad
a few days in advance 'to go'
then don't add the pumpkin
seeds to the portion of salad
in your lunch box until just
before you set out to work
so that they stay crunchy.

This salad is full of flavour and skin-loving omega-3
goodness. The courgette ribbons are coated in
delicious pine-nut-and-basil pesto and mixed with
toasted pumpkin seeds and caramelised butternut
squash – lots of healthy fats and natural oils. You
can make this in advance and the courgette ribbons
will 'wilt' making them more pasta-like in texture.

Preheat the oven to 190°C/170°C fan/gas 5. Spread
the butternut squash out in a roasting tin, drizzle with
the olive oil, add a pinch of salt and place in the oven
to roast for around 30 minutes until well caramelised
and soft.

For the tamari-caramelised pumpkin seeds, mix
the ingredients together in a bowl and spread out
in a baking tray lined with parchment paper or foil.
Pop into the oven to roast for around 5 minutes,
checking frequently and tossing once or twice to
ensure they don't burn. Allow to cool before using,
so they crisp up a bit more.

Meanwhile, make the pesto by adding all ingredients
to a food processor and processing until smooth, then
set aside. Using a vegetable peeler, peel the courgettes
into ribbons and place in a serving bowl.

To assemble the salad, pour the pesto over the
courgette ribbons and toss so they're all really well
coated, then add the roasted butternut squash and
scatter with the pumpkin seeds.

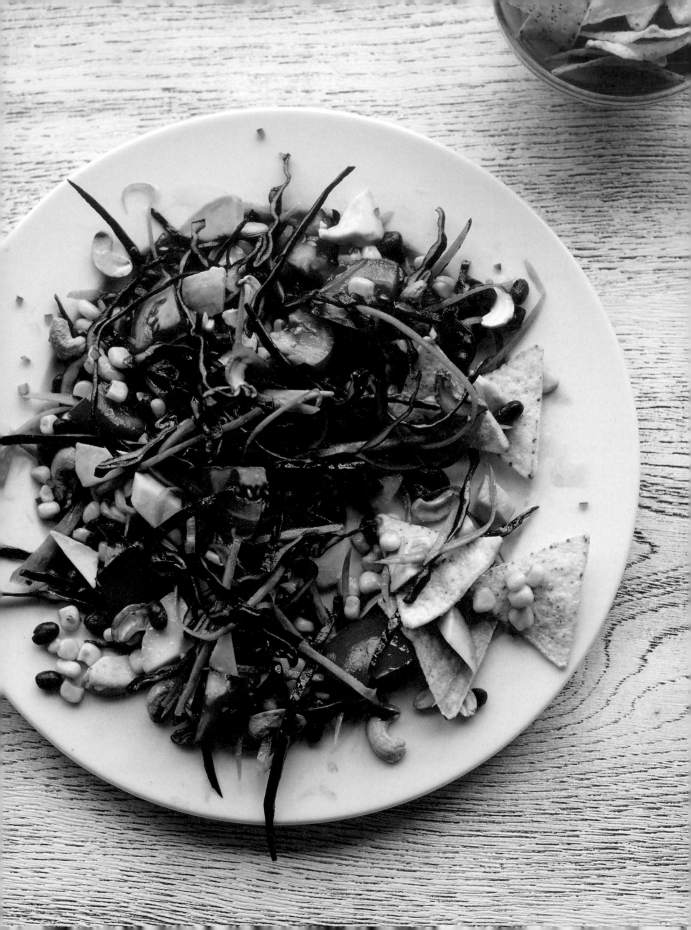

Mexican slaw with tamari vinaigrette and roasted cashews

SERVES 4

2 carrots, peeled and cut
 into matchsticks
12 cherry tomatoes, halved
6 red cabbage leaves,
 chopped
1 x 200g tin of sweetcorn
1 x 400g tin of black beans
1 big handful fresh coriander,
 chopped
100g (¾ cup) raw cashews,
 chopped in half
1 avocado, peeled,
 stoned and sliced
1 large bag (4 cups) of
 lightly salted gluten-free
 tortilla chips

Dressing
Juice of 1 lime
2 tablespoons tamari
5 tablespoons extra-virgin
 olive oil
⅓ red chilli, deseeded
 and finely diced
1 tablespoon peeled and
 grated fresh root ginger

TIP

If you're making this salad
a few days in advance 'to go'
then omit the avocado,
adding it to your lunch box,
along with a portion of the
salad, the night before and
storing in the fridge. Take
a small bag of gluten-free
tortilla chips with you to
accompany the salad.

This simple slaw is bursting with flavour and vibrant colour, making it an absolute feast for the senses. I'm a big fan of textures that mesh together perfectly – the crispy crunch of the carrots and red cabbage going like a dream with the creamy cubes of avocado. It's also a really easy and inexpensive recipe to prepare, so I often make quite a big batch as it keeps well in the fridge and is great paired alongside just about everything.

◇◇◇◇◇◇◇◇◇◇◇◇◇◇◇◇◇◇◇◇◇◇◇◇◇◇◇◇◇◇◇◇◇◇

Preheat the oven to 180°C/160°C fan/gas 4. Place the prepared vegetables in a large bowl with the coriander. Drain and rinse the sweetcorn and beans and add to bowl.

Tip the cashews onto a baking tray and toast in the oven for around 5 minutes or until light brown, shaking the tin once or twice to ensure they don't burn. Remove from the oven and add to the bowl, along with the avocado, and toss together.

For the dressing, simply mix all the ingredients together, stir well and pour over the slaw. Toss together well and top with the tortilla chips to serve.

Roasted vegetable salad with a hummus dressing

SERVES 2

2 red peppers, deseeded
1 yellow pepper, deseeded
1 red onion, peeled
1 courgette
2 sweet potatoes, peeled (optional)
12 cherry tomatoes, halved
2 tablespoons olive oil
Pinch of salt
2 Little Gem lettuces
1 avocado, peeled, stoned and cubed

Hummus dressing
1 tablespoon hummus (to make your own, see page 165)
2 tablespoons extra-virgin olive oil
Juice of 1 lemon
1 teaspoon tamari
2 teaspoons raw honey, agave or pure maple syrup

TIPS

I always make a batch of roasted vegetables to add to salads during the week, a great way to spice up some nutrient-rich greens!

If you're making this salad a few days in advance 'to go' then omit the lettuce and avocado, adding them to your lunch box, along with a portion of the salad, the night before and storing in the fridge.

The combination of the sweet roasted vegetables with the crunchy shredded lettuce and creamy hummus dressing is truly sensational. I'm a complete hummus fiend, so I'm always looking for new ways to use it, and this dressing is a winner.

◇◇◇◇◇◇◇◇◇◇◇◇◇◇◇◇◇◇◇◇◇◇◇◇◇◇◇◇

Preheat the oven to 190°C/170°C fan/gas 5. Chop the peppers, red onion and courgette into medium-sized chunks, and the sweet potatoes (if using) into similar-sized cubes. Place in a roasting tin with the tomatoes, then drizzle with olive oil, add a pinch of salt and roast in the oven for around 45 minutes.

Meanwhile, shred the lettuces by chopping each one finely from the end, and place in a serving bowl. Make the dressing by adding all the ingredients to a separate bowl and stirring together until smooth.

When the vegetables are well roasted, allow to cool slightly before placing in the salad bowl with the shredded lettuce. Pour over the hummus dressing and toss everything thoroughly together, then serve topped with the avocado.

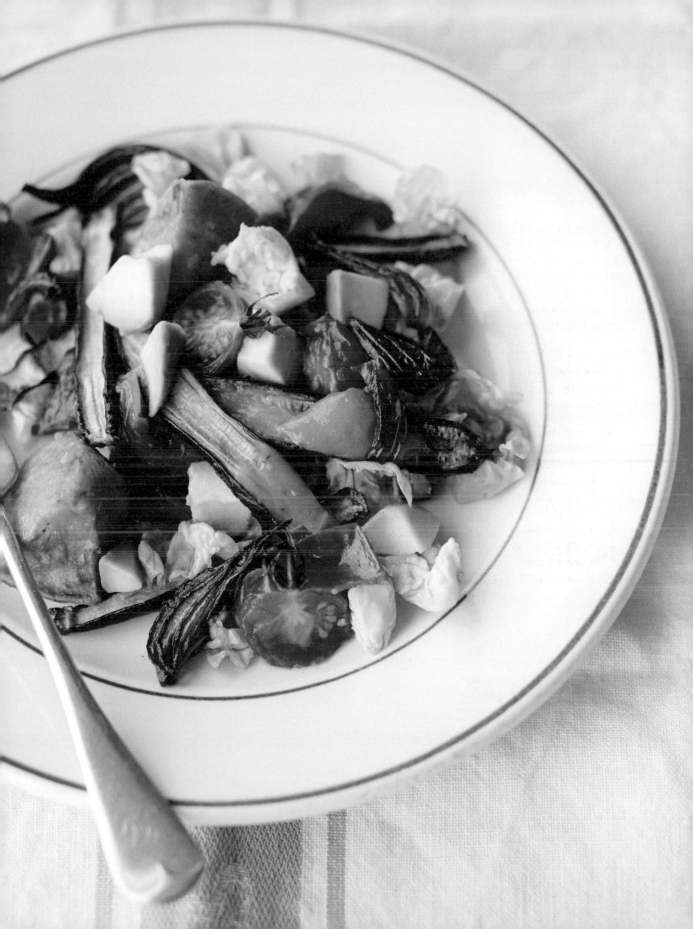

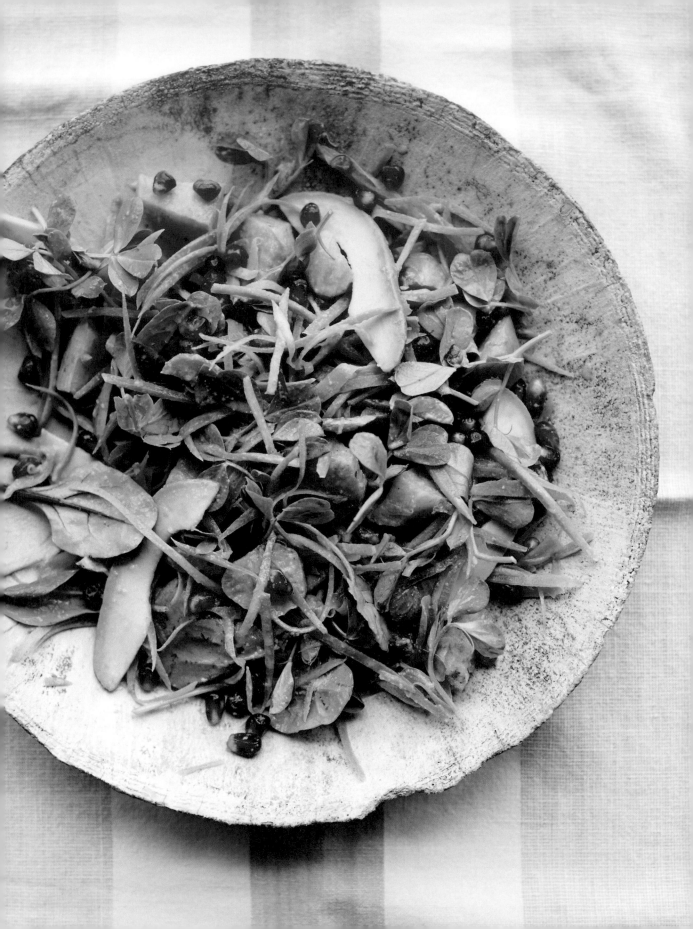

Baby leaf, pomegranate, avocado and sweet potato salad with an orange dressing

SERVES 1

1 medium-sized sweet
   potato, peeled and cut
   into small cubes
2 tablespoons olive oil
Pinch of salt
1 avocado, peeled and stoned
1 carrot, peeled
5 handfuls of baby leaf salad
45g (¼ cup) pomegranate
   seeds, plus extra to garnish

Orange dressing
4 tablespoons fresh orange
   juice (squeezed from
   an orange!)
1 teaspoon apple cider
   vinegar
2 teaspoon tamari
1 tablespoon tahini
   or almond butter
1 tablespoon water

TIP

If you're making this salad
a few days in advance 'to go'
then omit the avocado,
adding it to your lunch box,
along with a portion of the
salad, the night before and
storing in the fridge.

The main appeal of this salad lies in the simple, clear-cut flavours. Each ingredient adds a different taste and texture, from the caramelised sweet potato and zingily sweet pomegranate to the creamy avocado and crunchy carrot. They all combine to create a wonderfully satisfying superfood salad.

Preheat the oven to 190°C/170°C fan/gas 5. Spread the sweet potato in a roasting tin, drizzle with the olive oil and sprinkle with the salt, then place in the oven to roast for around 30 minutes or until soft.

Meanwhile, make the dressing. Combine all the ingredients in a bowl and stir quickly for a minute until smooth. Next grate the carrot and cut the avocado flesh into cubes or slices.

Place the salad leaves in a serving bowl with the grated carrot, avocado and pomegranate seeds, add the dressing and toss well so all the leaves are coated. Top with the roasted sweet potato and garnish with a sprinkling of pomegranate seeds.

Lemon-infused wild rice with parsley, dried apricots and pistachios

SERVES 4

80g (½ cup) raw pistachio
kernels
125g (⅔ cup) wild rice
(I buy a mixed bag of
brown basmati, red
Camargue and wild rice)
315ml (1⅓ cups) boiling
water
100g (⅔ cup) dried apricots
(unsulphured)
2 large handfuls of rocket
1 handful of fresh mint,
finely chopped
1 handful of fresh parsley,
finely chopped
Juice of 1 lemon

Dressing
2 tablespoons extra-virgin
olive oil
½ clove garlic, peeled
and crushed
Salt and pepper

TIP

If you're making this salad
a few days in advance 'to go'
then omit the rocket and fresh
herbs, adding them to your
lunch box, along with a
portion of the salad, the
night before and storing
in the fridge.

Wild rice infused with lemon juice and mixed with parsley and mint makes an alkaline combo that tastes incredible as well as being really good for you. What's more, the nuttiness of the pistachios and the burst of sweetness from the apricots really complement the citrusy flavour running through the dish. I'm always preparing great bowlfuls of this salad for lunch parties, as everyone loves it and it's more cost-effective made in bigger batches. A real win-win!

◇◇◇◇◇◇◇◇◇◇◇◇◇◇◇◇◇◇◇◇◇◇◇◇◇◇◇◇◇◇◇◇◇

Preheat the oven to 180°C/160°C fan/gas 4. Spread the pistachios on a baking tray, place in the oven and toast for around 7 minutes, checking on them frequently and tossing once or twice to ensure they don't burn. Take them out and chop into small chunks.

Meanwhile, tip the rice into a saucepan and add the water. Bring to the boil, then reduce the heat and simmer for 30–40 minutes until tender and fluffy and all the water has been absorbed. Drain, rinsing with cold water.

While the rice is cooking, put the apricots in a bowl, cover with boiling water and leave to soak for 2 minutes. Drain and chop into small pieces.

Place the cooked rice in a bowl with the rice, rocket, pistachios, apricots and chopped herbs. For the dressing combine the olive oil, lemon, crushed garlic and salt stir and pour over the rice mixing well. Then serve!

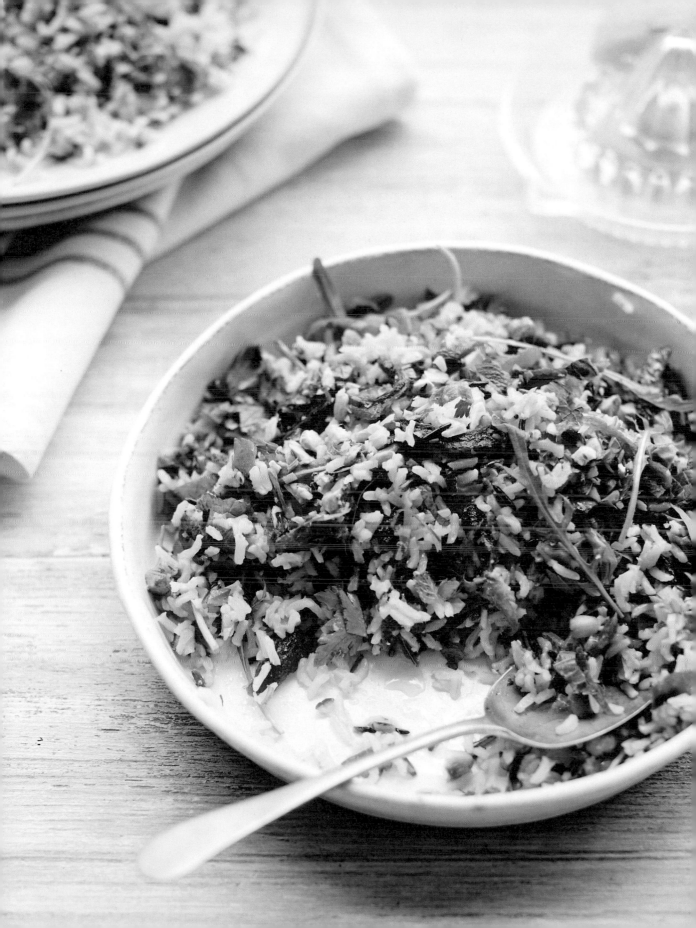

Brown rice pasta salad with avocado, rocket and pesto vinaigrette

SERVES 2

110g (1 cup) brown rice
  fusilli or penne
Pinch of salt
1 large or 2 small avocados,
  peeled, stoned and cubed
3 handfuls of rocket

Pesto vinaigrette
2 heaped tablespoons pesto
  (to make your own,
  see page 97)
4 tablespoons extra-virgin
  olive oil (you may need
  more or less depending
  on the consistency of
  the pesto)
Juice of ½ lemon

TIP
If you're making this salad
a few days in advance 'to go'
then omit the avocado and
rocket, adding them to your
lunch box, along with a
portion of the salad, the
night before and storing
in the fridge.

This recipe happened completely by chance, made with store-cupboard basics and the only fresh ingredients that I had to hand. It turned out to be one of my favourite recipes in the book. The brown rice pasta is paired with peppery rocket, creamy cubes of avocado and an amazingly delicious pesto vinaigrette. The perfect energising salad.

◇◇◇◇◇◇◇◇◇◇◇◇◇◇◇◇◇◇◇◇◇◇◇◇◇◇◇◇◇◇◇◇◇

Cook the pasta in boiling, salted water following the instructions on the packet. This normally takes around 10 minutes. While it is cooking, make the vinaigrette by simply combining all the ingredients in a bowl.

Once the pasta is cooked, rinse with cold water and drain, then add to a bowl with the avocado cubes and rocket. Drizzle over the pesto vinaigrette and toss together until everything is well coated, then serve!

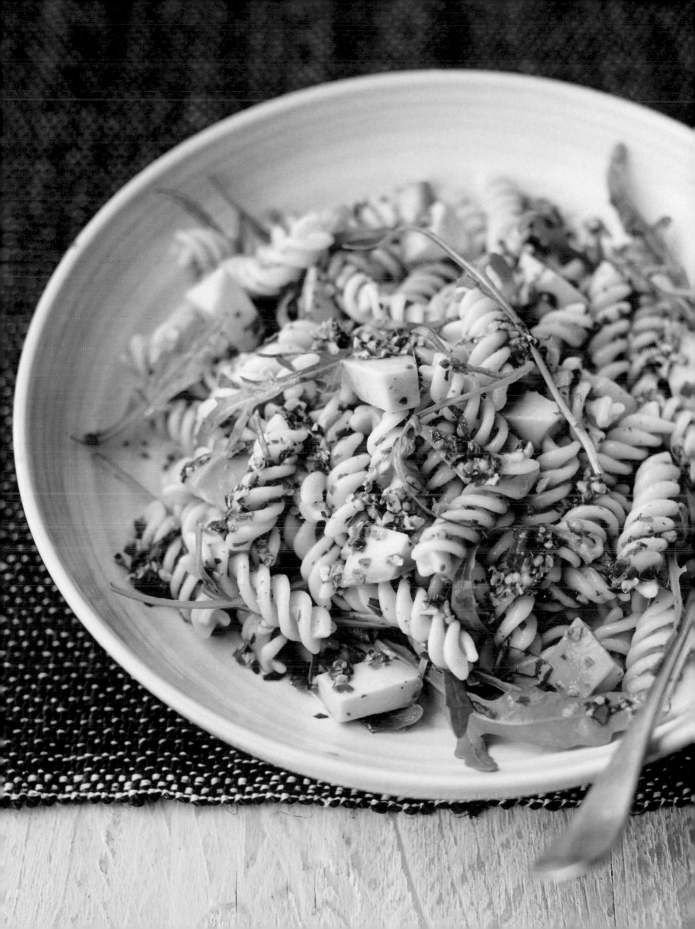

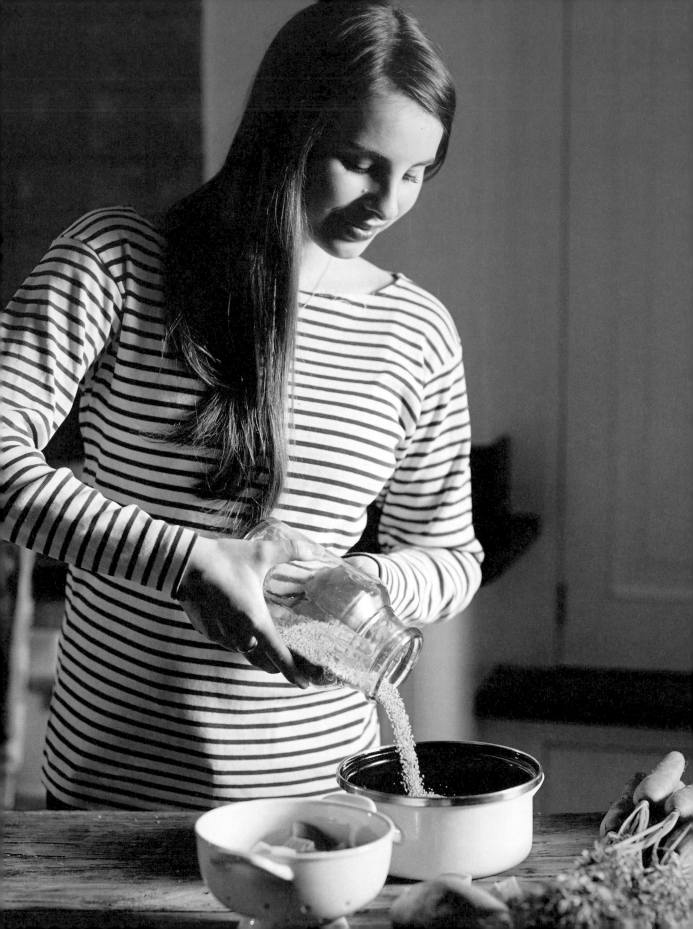

Sunday prep

While it's all very well saying healthy eating is easy, what do you do when you're out and about or having to eat lunch at work? This is actually the most important meal to prepare for, as it can often be the hardest time to maintain a good diet. Convenience stores and fast-food cafés and restaurants are plentiful, and if you're in a rush and need to grab lunch, you can all too often be lured through their doors into a delicious, though extremely unhealthy trap. The way to resist is via a little bit of forward preparation – about an hour at the weekend (you'll get quicker with practice!) and you'll have made a selection of great cooked wholefoods you can assemble into a packed lunch for each day of the week. On a Sunday night, I always prepare a few batches of different foods and leave them on a shelf in my fridge ready for a pick-and-mix lunch I can whip up in 5 minutes every weeknight for the following day. I like to make a really good range of foods so I never get bored. This section is all about showing you how to make really tasty, affordable meals for when you're on the go. I've listed everything you need to buy or make in advance. The only special equipment you'll need is a range of airtight plastic boxes for storing the food and for your lunch each day. Tupperware will be your new best friend!

Roasted sweet potato
4 medium-sized sweet
   potatoes, peeled and
   cut into small cubes
2 tablespoons olive oil
Generous pinch of salt

Spicy seed mix
35g (¼ cup) mixed seeds
   (such as sesame, pumpkin
   and sunflower)
½ tablespoon tamari
Pinch of chilli flakes

Lentils
200g (1 cup) dried lentils
   (such as beluga, Puy
   or green lentils)
475ml (2 cups) vegetable
   stock (made with a stock
   cube or bouillon powder)

Quinoa
250g (1½ cups) quinoa
700ml (3 cups) boiling water
Juice of 1 lemon
Pinch of salt

Roasted sweet potato
Preheat the oven to 190°C/170°C fan/gas 5. Spread the sweet potatoes out in a roasting tin, drizzle with the olive oil and add a big pinch of salt. Put in the oven to roast for around 30 minutes. Remove from the oven and allow to cool before placing in an airtight plastic box and storing in the fridge.

Spicy seed mix
While the oven is on, make the seed mix by simply mixing all the ingredients together, placing in a small roasting tin or baking tray and roasting for around 3 minutes. Check once or twice and shake the tin to ensure they don't burn. Remove from the oven and leave to cool before tipping into a clean jar or small airtight plastic container.

Lentils
Next put the lentils into a saucepan and add the stock. Bring to the boil, then reduce to a simmer and cook for about 30 minutes. Drain well and allow to cool before putting into another plastic box for storing in the fridge.

Quinoa
Meanwhile, place the quinoa in another saucepan and add the water. Bring back up to the boil, then reduce to a simmer and cook for 15–20 minutes or until soft and fluffy, adding more water if needed. Once cooked, add the lemon juice and a pinch of salt, then allow to cool before transferring to a plastic box and placing in the fridge.

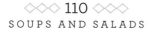

Beetroot, carrot and sultana slaw
4 beetroots, peeled
4 carrots, peeled
50g (⅓ cup) sultanas
Juice of 1 lemon
Pinch of salt

Kale salad with tahini dressing
5 tablespoons tahini
5 tablespoons tamari
Juice of 3 lemons
5 tablespoons water
3 x 180g bags of kale,
    thick stems removed
Seeds of 1 pomegranate

Extras
1 large tub of hummus
    (to make it yourself,
    see page 165)
3 avocados, peeled,
    stoned and sliced
1 x 140g bag of rocket

TIP

Any fresh extras that go
off quickly, such as slices
of avocado or handfuls of
fresh lettuce, are best added
to your lunch box the night
before (then stored in the
fridge) or just before
you leave.

Beetroot, carrot and sultana slaw
Now prepare the beetroots and carrots by grating
them both into a plastic container and mixing with
the sultanas, lemon juice and salt. Place in the fridge.

Kale salad with tahini dressing
Mix together all the ingredients for the tahini dressing
in a large bowl and add the kale. Work the dressing
into the kale with your hands (as if massaging them)
for a few minutes until the leaves are completely
wilted, add the pomegranate seeds and put in another
container before storing in the fridge.

Picking and mixing
For your 'evening prep' (each week night), you could
add to your lunch box: a generous amount of the kale
salad, beetroot and carrot slaw, roasted sweet potato,
quinoa and lentils, a good dollop of hummus, some
cubes of avocado, a few rocket leaves and a sprinkling
of seeds. Delicious! This is just an example, of course
– you can add whatever you please from the selection
above. I love to mix it up so it **really does** change
every day.

SWITCH IT UP

The different options don't just end here! Rather than
restrict yourself to the salads I've suggested above, why
not swap one or more of them for something from the main
'Salads' section (see pages 92–106)? Each of them can be
made ahead for the week, just like the other dishes here,
and stored in an airtight plastic container, with certain fresh
ingredients added at the last minute. You can even take the
soups (see pages 87–91) to go, especially when the weather
gets chillier and you fancy something warming. Just as I do,
you can make up a big batch as part of your Sunday prep and
store it in fridge, then heat up a single portion shortly before
you leave for work, pouring it into a flask to take with you.

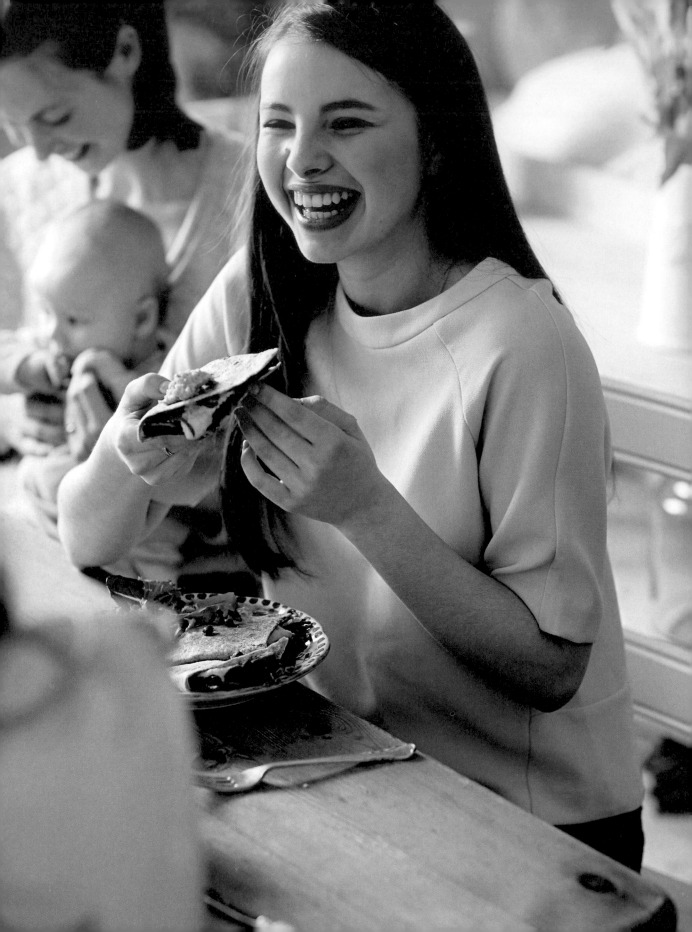

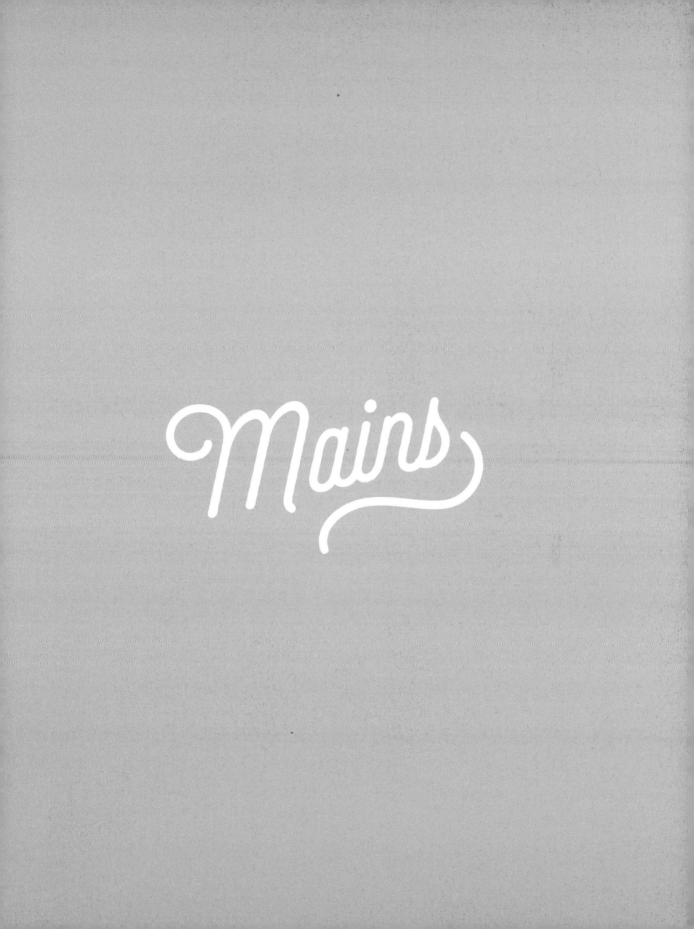

Mains

A healthy dinner can be the last thing on your mind after a long day at work.

I've therefore devised all these recipes with both time and the occasion in mind – from one-pot dishes and 15-minute meals for a casual get-together to slightly longer (no more than 45 minutes) fancier recipes for more formal gatherings. I've got you covered for whatever life throws at you! All about nourishment and comfort, these dishes are intended to make you feel good from the inside out, and give you exactly what you need to fully recharge the batteries.

The first section in this chapter is the 'I'm too tired to wash up' main. Admittedly this is the category I often fall into! It's brilliant for lazy weekends or those evenings when you just want to collapse completely. These one-pot wonders (see pages 115–120) really do require very little effort all round. The recipes include some of the most comforting dishes in the chapter, like my Creamy one-pot pasta (see page 119).

Next you have the 'I can't be bothered' main, for when you're just too tired or rushed off your feet and need something that can be knocked up in only 15 minutes. It includes favourites like my Hummus and black bean quesadillas (see page 130). Despite being 'fast food', they're delicious, giving a healthy twist on some much-loved takeaway dishes.

Of course, there's the middle ground, the 'I can make a little effort' main. Pages 131–142 are full of recipes that take up to 45 minutes to make, but are still fairly speedy and, as always, don't need all that many ingredients. My top favourites are the Vegan enchiladas and Sweet potato and spinach dhal, accompanied by a gluten-free naan bread, made from chickpea flour (see pages 134 and 141–142).

Occasionally you may need the 'I want to make a good impression' main, for which you can turn to pages 144–156. These recipes take anywhere between 45 minutes to just over an hour, but even this is usually just the cooking time, not so much the prep. Including some of my favourite dishes – such as the scrumptious Spicy squash and black bean burgers (page 146) – these are the ones I love to make to show people just how delicious healthy vegan food can be.

Finally, there's the 'I need to use these ingredients up' main, which can sometimes be the most delicious! In 'How to Make a Balance Bowl' (see pages 158–159), I've given instructions on how to assemble a delicious, nourishing meal from a whole range of different foods or whatever you may have in the fridge.

So, whatever time of day it is, whoever (and however many) you're catering for and whatever ingredients you prefer or happen to have, there'll be something in this chapter that's perfect for you!

Baked sweet potatoes with miso beluga lentils and mushrooms

SERVES 2

2 large or 4 small-to-medium-sized sweet potatoes (unpeeled)
240ml (1 cup) water
1 tablespoon miso
100g (½ cup) dried beluga lentils
150g (1½ cups) sliced white mushrooms
1 handful of chopped parsley

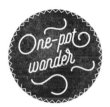

Oven-baked sweet potatoes are one of the easiest things to cook – the most work required is to preheat the oven! This makes them ideal for easy recipes, as all you need is a delicious filling to liven things up.

Preheat the oven to 190°C/170°C fan/gas 5. Score each sweet potato and pop in the oven to bake for 35–45 minutes.

Meanwhile, place the water and miso in a pan, bring to the boil and add the beluga lentils and sliced mushrooms. Lower the heat to a simmer and cook for 20–25 minutes until the lentils are tender.

Check on your sweet potatoes and, if they 'give' when you squeeze them gently, take them out of the oven, slice each in half lengthways and place on individual plates. Mix the parsley in with the mushrooms and lentils and spoon on top of the sweet potatoes. Serve with a dollop of hummus (to make your own, see page 165) on the side.

SWITCH IT UP

If you can't find beluga lentils, why not try quinoa (cooked in the same way but for 15–20 minutes)? I also love switching up the miso in this recipe for a tablespoon of tamari.

GREEDY FOR GOODNESS?

If you love your greens as much as I do, why not wilt some kale or spinach into the lentils shortly before they have finished cooking?

Pho courgette noodle soup

SERVES 4

2 tablespoons olive oil
1 medium-sized red onion,
    peeled and finely chopped
1 tablespoon peeled and
    grated fresh root ginger
325g (3¼ cups) sliced
    white mushrooms
130g (1¾ cups) sliced
    shiitake mushrooms
1 litre (4¼ cups) vegetable
    stock (made with a stock
    cube or bouillon powder)
220g tenderstem broccoli
    spears, chopped
150g (1½ cups) baby corn
80g (1½ cups) spinach
4 courgettes, spiralised
    or peeled into strips with
    a vegetable peeler

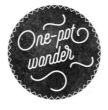

I love a hearty bowl of noodle soup, so comforting and full of nourishment, and this is my take on the classic Vietnamese- style pho. Instead of wheat-based noodles, I've used ones made from 'spiralised' courgettes, which work really well in this dish as well as being better for you. If you don't have a spiraliser, I'd highly recommend investing in one – they're one of the most affordable kitchen tools and something you'll love using. (For more information, see page 12.) I use mine all the time – daily, in fact!

Drizzle the olive oil into a pan and, when the oil is hot, add the onion and ginger. Sauté over a medium-high heat for 5–7 minutes until fragrant and the onion starts to caramelise. Tip in the mushrooms and sauté again for a further 4–5 minutes.

Now pour in the vegetable stock and add the broccoli, baby corn, spinach and spiralised courgette 'noodles'. Bring to the boil and then lower the heat and leave to simmer for a further 5 minutes until everything is cooked. Pour into bowls and serve!

SWITCH IT UP

I love the courgette noodles in this dish, but why not try buckwheat or brown rice noodles instead? You can also play around with the vegetables: replacing the ones in this recipe with carrots, kale and steamed squash would work a treat!

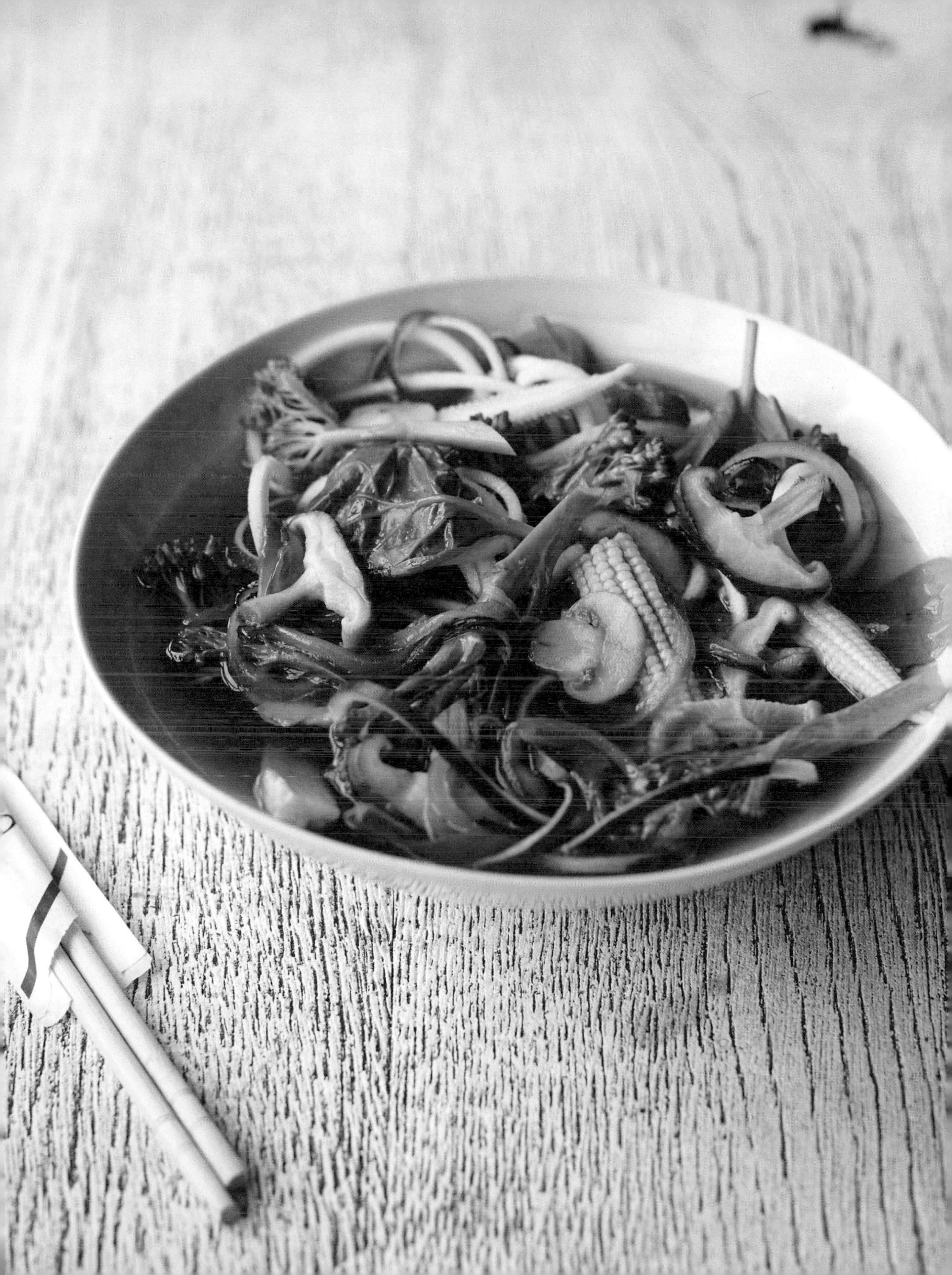

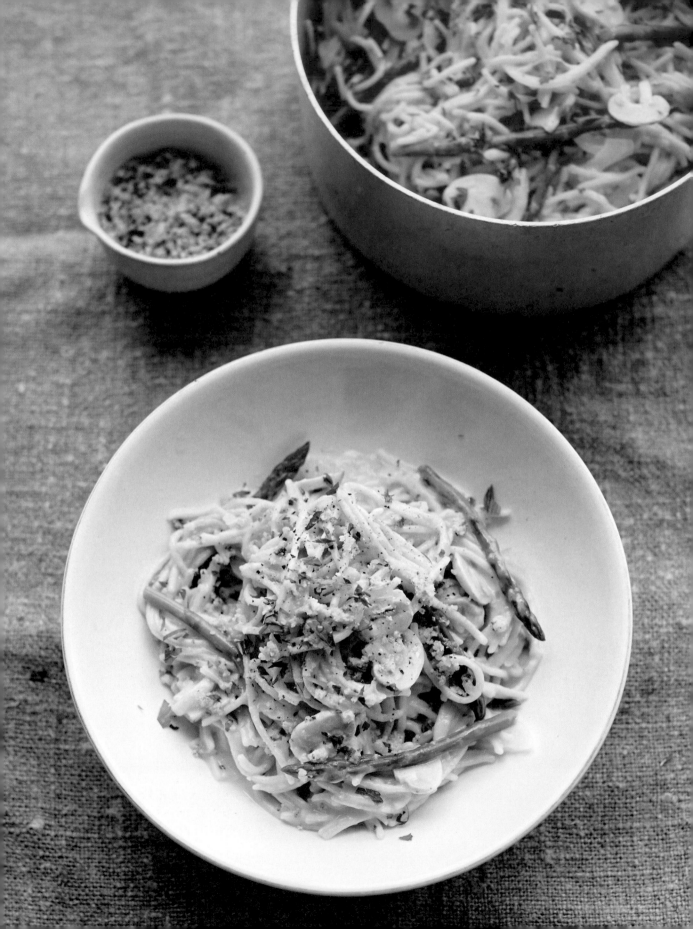

Creamy one-pot pasta

SERVES 4

1 litre (4¼ cups) vegetable
    stock (made with a stock
    cube or bouillon powder)
400g dried brown rice
    spaghetti
1 small onion, peeled
    and finely chopped
450g asparagus spears,
    chopped into 5cm lengths
325g (3¼ cups) sliced
    white mushrooms
2 cloves of garlic, peeled
    and finely chopped
2 tablespoons olive oil
60ml (¼ cup) coconut cream
2 teaspoons freshly grated
    lemon zest
1 small handful of fresh
    parsley, chopped, plus
    extra for sprinkling
2 tablespoons nutritional
    yeast (optional)
Brazil nut Parmesan, for
    sprinkling (see page
    150 – optional)
Salt and pepper

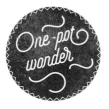

This recipe for a one-pot pasta is pure genius ... if I do say so myself. This isn't (only) because it is really tasty, but because of the sheer ease of it. You simply pop all ingredients in one pan and let it cook away. Not only do you get a great result, but minimal effort is required! The other benefit of cooking it all in one pot is the way the pasta absorbs all the flavour.

Add the stock to a pan with the spaghetti, onion, asparagus, mushrooms and garlic. Season with salt and pepper and drizzle over the olive oil. Place over a high heat and when it starts to bubble, set your stopwatch or timer for 7 minutes, leaving the mixture to cook at a gentle boil. During this time you need to move the spaghetti strands around regularly to ensure they don't get stuck together.

After the 7 minutes, add the coconut cream, lemon zest, parsley and nutritional yeast (if using). Toss all the ingredients together in the pan for a further 2–3 minutes until the pasta is tender and ready to eat and the liquid has reduced to a creamy sauce. Remove the pan from the hob and leave it to cool down for a few minutes before dividing between individual bowls to serve. Garnish with parsley and some brazil nut Parmesan, if you wish, then tuck in!

SWITCH IT UP

While I love this creamy combo, you can switch it up by having a tomato sauce made with passata and basil to replace the coconut cream. Feel free to use other vegetables too. Why not try some tenderstem broccoli or spinach instead of the asparagus?

Coconut rice with a mango and avocado salsa

SERVES 3–4

240ml (1 cup) full-fat
    coconut milk
350ml (1½ cups) boiling
    water
150g (¾ cup) brown rice
1 teaspoon peeled and finely
    chopped fresh root ginger
Juice of 1 lemon
Salt and pepper

Mango and avocado salsa
1 mango, peeled, stoned
    and diced
2 avocados, peeled,
    stoned and diced
1 red pepper, deseeded
    and chopped
Juice of 1 lime
1 handful of fresh coriander,
    finely chopped

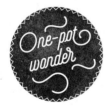

I've always loved coconut rice and the tropical flavours it marries so well with. Topping it with my favourite mango and avocado salsa is truly a match made in heaven. This dish is full of healthy fats, giving you constant energy and a glowing skin – a killer combination!

Pour the coconut milk and water into a pan and add the rice, ginger, lemon juice and a pinch of salt. Bring to the boil, then reduce the heat and simmer for up to 40 minutes, or until the rice is cooked. Stir every so often, to ensure it doesn't catch on the bottom of the pan, and add a touch more water if needed.

Meanwhile, make the mango and avocado salsa by adding all ingredients to a bowl and mixing together, seasoning with salt and pepper to taste. Tip the coconut rice into a serving dish and pour the salsa on top. Enjoy!

GREEDY FO R GOODNESS?

This dish has a trifecta of stunning colours, and contains so many delicious and healthy ingredients – a winner on every front! If you want to up the goodness factor, you can also add 1 sweet potato, peeled, diced and roasted (see page 110), to the coconut rice mixture. Take one bite and prepare to be amazed!

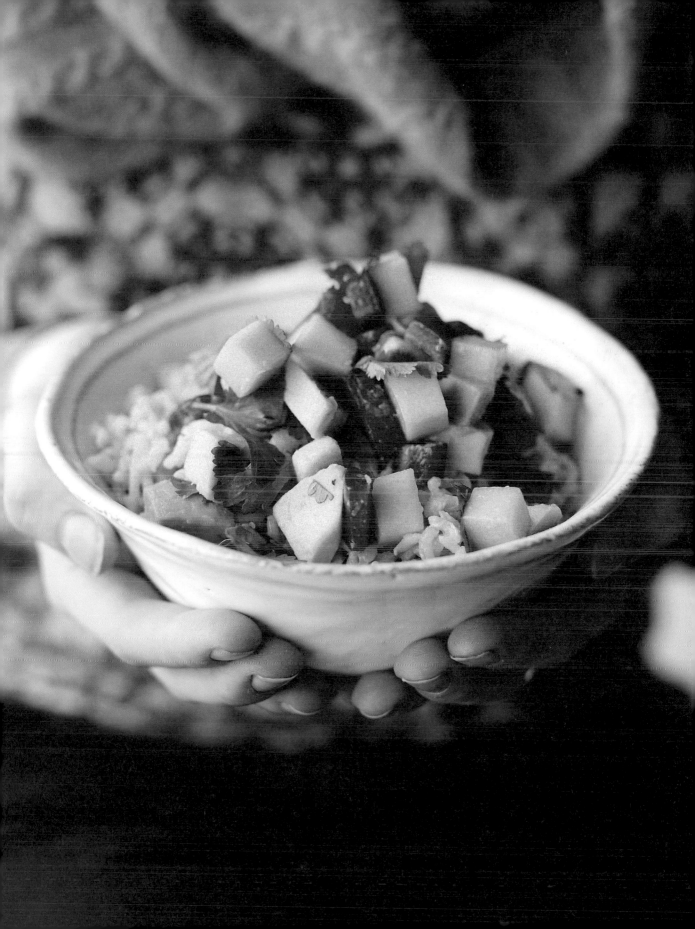

Pad Thai

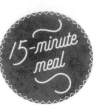

SERVES 4

6 courgettes
3 carrots, peeled
5 asparagus spears,
    very thinly sliced
2 red peppers, deseeded
    and thinly sliced

Tamari-roasted almonds
50g (⅓ cup) whole almonds
1 tablespoon tamari
1 tablespoon water

Sauce
3 Medjool dates, pitted
    and chopped
2 cloves of garlic, peeled
    and crushed
1 thumbnail-sized knob
    of fresh root ginger,
    peeled and grated
240ml (1 cup) full-fat
    coconut milk
80g (⅓ cup) almond butter
Juice of 1 lime
2 tablespoons tamari

TIP
For the sauce, make sure
you buy a standard brand of
coconut milk. Some specialist
brands can be very thin and
watery, and we don't want
a watery sauce!

This 'raw' take on the classic pad Thai is full
of fabulous flavours, using ingredients that both
taste wonderful and do your body so much good.
The sauce is a powerhouse in its own right, and
I'm constantly devising new recipes to use it in.
Topped off with tamari-roasted almonds, the
layers of flavour and texture are never-ending!
I'm pretty obsessed with these delicious almonds;
they're so addictive that I find I have to make
double the batch as otherwise they're gone
before we've even sat down!

Preheat the oven to 180°C/160°C fan/gas 4. To make
the tamari-roasted almonds, combine the tamari and
water in a bowl, add the almonds and coat well in the
liquid. Tip into a baking tray, spreading out evenly,
then place in the oven to roast for 2–3 minutes, until
the liquid has dissolved. Remove from the oven
and set aside.

Next spiralise the courgettes and carrots with a
spiraliser if you have one (see page 12) or peel them
into fine ribbons with a vegetable peeler if you don't.
To prepare the sauce, simply chuck all the sauce
ingredients into a blender and blend!

To assemble the dish, place all the prepared
vegetables into a large mixing bowl, add the
tamari-roasted almonds, pour in the sauce and
toss well together. Plate up and enjoy!

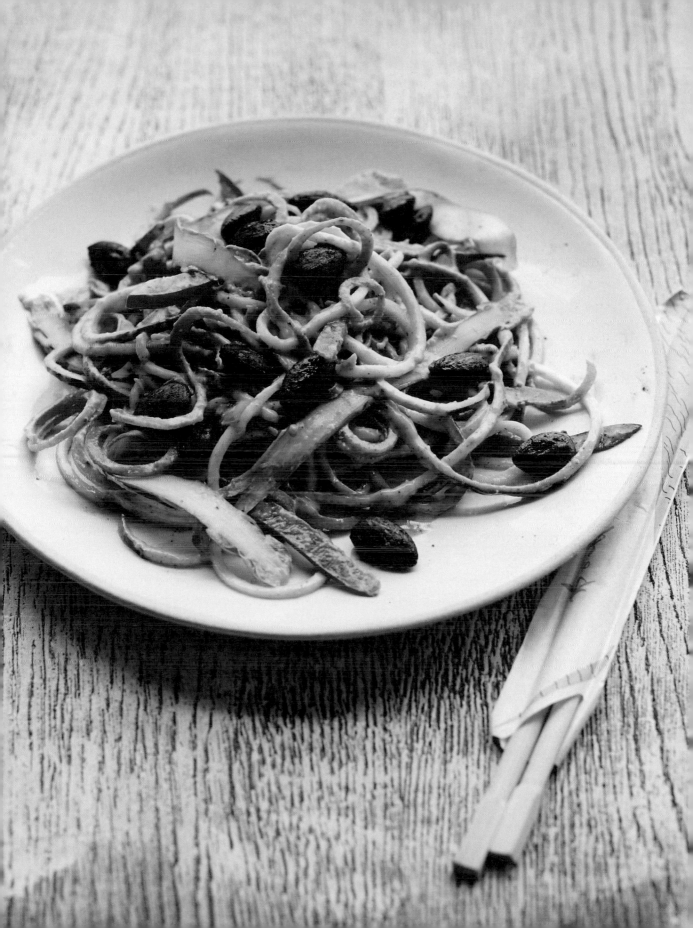

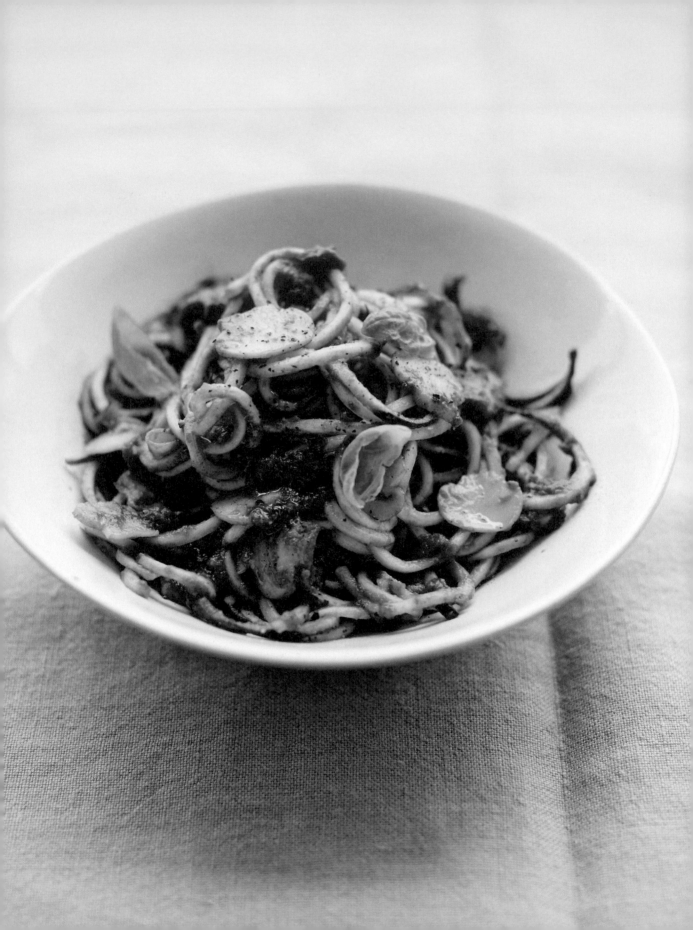

Courgette noodles with a sun-dried tomato sauce and sautéed mushrooms

SERVES 2

5 courgettes
1 tablespoon olive oil
150g (1½ cups) sliced
    white mushrooms

Sun-dried tomato sauce
60g (1 cup) sun-dried
    tomatoes
1 tablespoon extra-virgin
    olive oil
2 plum tomatoes (fresh
    or tinned), chopped
1 handful of fresh basil
½ clove of garlic, peeled

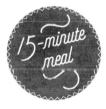

The combination of courgettes, sun-dried tomatoes, toasted pine nuts and sautéed mushrooms makes for the perfect meal. Courgette noodles are the easiest thing to prepare if you have a spiraliser (see page 12), though you can peel them into fine strips with a vegetable peeler if you don't. They'll taste equally delicious!

First spiralise the courgettes, or peel them into fine strips using a vegetable peeler, and add to a bowl.

For the sauce, simply add everything to a blender and blend until smooth. Pour the sauce into the bowl with the courgettes, or heat it through in a saucepan and then pour it into the bowl and mix until combined.

Finally, add the olive oil to a pan, followed by the mushrooms, and sauté over a medium heat for 4–5 minutes until soft, then add to the bowl!

GREEDY FOR GOODNESS?
If you want to make your sun-dried tomato sauce even more awesome than it already is, add 1 teaspoon turmeric. It's highly anti-inflammatory!

Tomato and chilli stir-fry with lemon-infused quinoa

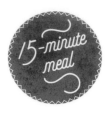

15-minute meal

SERVES 2

85g (½ cup) quinoa
240ml (1 cup) boiling water
2 tablespoons olive oil
1 teaspoon deseeded and finely chopped chilli (or to taste, depending on how hot you like it)
1 clove of garlic, peeled and finely chopped
1 red onion, peeled and finely chopped
2 red peppers, deseeded and sliced
2 courgettes, sliced
1 x 400g tin of chopped tomatoes
1 x 180g bag of spinach
Juice of 1 large or 2 small lemons
Pinch of salt

TIP

I'm a big fan of spicy food, but even I am shocked by how spicy this can sometimes be. This isn't the fault of the recipe – it's down to how strong the chilli is! Every chilli differs, so make sure you try a little bit of yours before you add it to the pan. Depending on how strong it is, you may want to add more or less.

This stir-fry is the perfect way to create a speedy but nourishing meal. Laden with veggie goodness, it's served over a warming bed of lemon-infused quinoa, which is not only a great source of plant-based protein, but tastes wonderful. Quinoa can be super-bland on its own, but in this dish it absorbs all the flavours from the tomato sauce and lemon, making it über-flavoursome and really moreish!

Add the quinoa and water to a saucepan and bring back up to the boil. Reduce the heat and simmer for 15–20 minutes or until fluffy, adding more water if needed.

Meanwhile, add the olive oil to another pan, followed by the chilli, garlic and onion, and sauté over a medium heat for about 5 minutes until the onion starts to caramelise. Now tip in the red peppers and courgettes and stir-fry for a further 10 minutes until the peppers are softened. Add the tinned tomatoes and spinach and cook until the spinach wilts and is piping hot.

The quinoa should now be done. Add the lemon juice and a pinch of salt, spoon into individual bowls and top with the tomato and chilli stir-fry!

SWITCH IT UP

Try substituting with your own favourites or with leftovers, keeping to similar quantities, and it should still be really yum. Try adding 1 peeled and diced sweet potato and 1 sliced aubergine to the mix, cooking the sweet potato first for around 5 minutes before adding the aubergine with the rest of the vegetables.

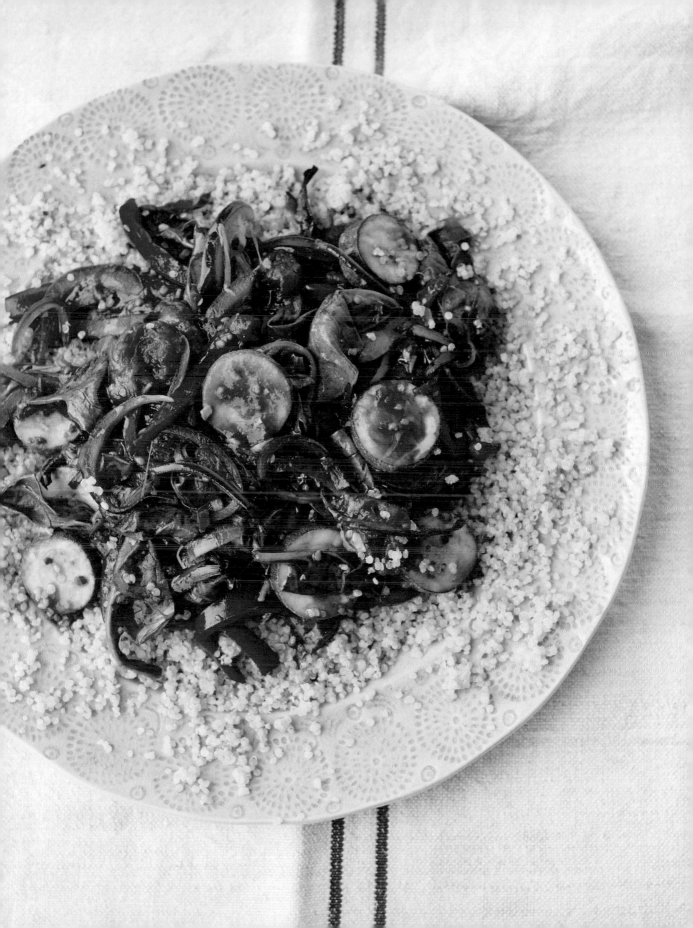

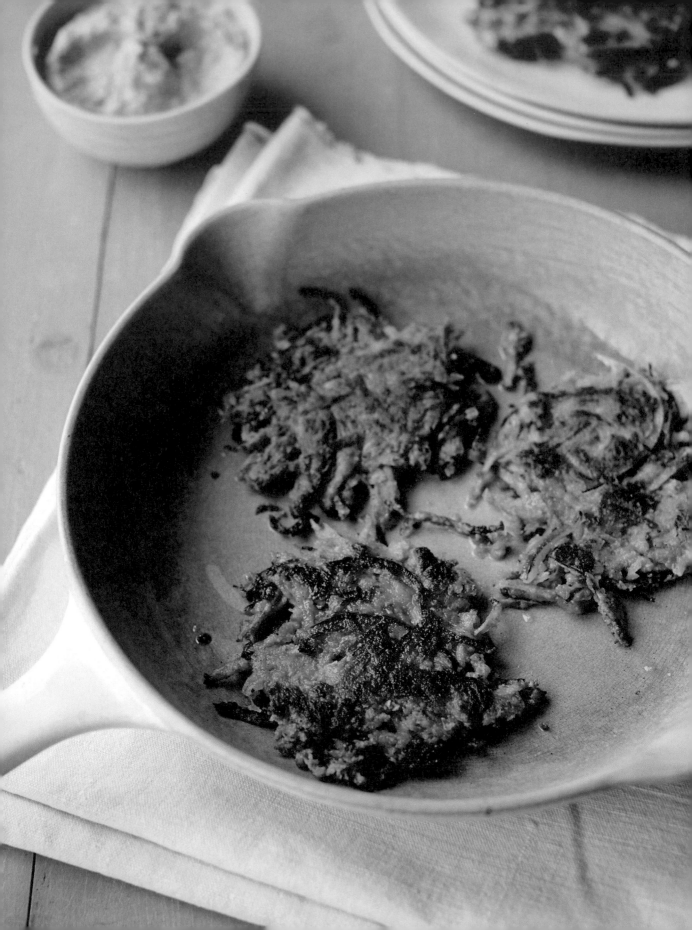

Spiced carrot, coriander and chickpea fritters

SERVES 2/MAKES 6 FRITTERS

4 medium-sized carrots, peeled and grated
½ red onion, peeled and chopped
50g (⅓ cup) tinned sweetcorn (optional)
90g (1 cup) chickpea flour (gram or besan flour)
1 handful of fresh coriander, roughly chopped
1 tablespoon olive oil, plus extra for frying
½ teaspoon ground cumin
Salt and pepper

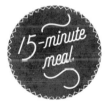

The word 'fritter' immediately conjures up deep-fried patties, swimming in grease, with an overwhelmingly oily taste. These are quite the reverse: light and deliciously healthy, yet hugely nourishing and totally satisfying. They're honestly so easy to make, too, and really eye-catching – if I do say so myself! The grated carrot, coriander and sweetcorn go incredibly well with the subtle flavour of the chickpea flour.

In a mixing bowl, combine all ingredients, mixing them together with a wooden spoon and adding salt and pepper to taste. Form the mixture into six fritters, each 8–9cm across.

Heat a little olive oil in a frying pan over a medium heat. Cooking 2–3 fritters at a time, fry for roughly 3 minutes on each side; they should be turning golden brown and cooked all the way through.

Serve with a generous dollop of my favourite hummus (see page 165) or, for a sneaky time-saver, simply buy some from the supermarket!

SWITCH IT UP

When I don't have carrots to hand, I love using grated beetroot or sweet potato instead. Either tastes super-delicious in these fritters, each with their own unique flavour. You can also substitute the chickpea flour for brown rice flour.

Hummus and black bean quesadillas

SERVES 1

2 gluten-free tortilla wraps
6 tablespoons hummus
(to make your own,
see page 165)
2 tablespoons olive oil

Black bean filling
1–2 tablespoons olive oil
1 red onion, peeled and
chopped
½ clove of garlic, peeled
and finely chopped
130g (½ cup) tinned
black beans
100g (2 cups) spinach
4 tablespoons passata

TIP
I love doing online shopping,
it's so much easier and I can
always get everything I want
in one place. Gluten-free
tortillas are a staple in my
household and I always
buy them online.

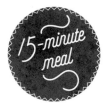

These quesadillas are the best, most delicious
way to create a speedy meal. They are so tasty, too,
that you honestly don't need any cheese! I'm also
obsessed with making quesadillas with leftover
cooked veggies; it's a really great way to use them
up. While this recipe is for just one person, it can
easily be multiplied to serve more.

Start by making the black bean filling. Add the
olive oil to a pan, followed by the onion and garlic,
and sauté over a medium heat for 5–7 minutes until
caramelised. Add the black beans to the pan with the
spinach and passata. Cook for a further 5–6 minutes
until nice and hot, and the spinach has wilted.

To assemble the quesadillas, spread one side of each
tortilla wrap with half the hummus. Spoon the black
bean mixture on top, fold the tortillas in half and cut
each down the middle.

Drizzle a little olive oil into a frying pan and add
two of the halved quesadillas. Cook over a medium
heat for 2–3 minutes, then flip over with a spatula
and repeat on the other side. Remove from the pan
and cook the other two quesadilla halves. Plate up
and serve!

SWITCH IT UP
If you've got a little more time, try adding one mashed sweet
potato in your quesadilla. It's so delicious, but, as you'll have
figured, will take you a little more than 15 minutes. It's best to
bake it first in the oven (preheated to 190°C/170°C fan/gas 5)
for 35–45 minutes and then just scoop out the soft flesh.

Chilli non-carne with spicy baked potato wedges and guacamole

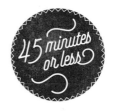

SERVES 4

Chilli non-carne
2 medium-sized sweet potatoes, peeled and cut into small cubes
2 tablespoons olive oil
1 onion, peeled and finely sliced
2 red peppers, deseeded and sliced
1 clove of garlic, peeled and crushed
1 red chilli, deseeded and finely chopped
¼ teaspoon ground cinnamon
1 teaspoon ground cumin
1 teaspoon cayenne pepper
2 x 400g tins of kidney beans, drained and rinsed
2 x 400g tins of chopped tomatoes
1 bunch of fresh coriander, chopped, to garnish

Spicy potato wedges (optional)
4–6 large sweet potatoes or white potatoes (unpeeled), cut into medium-sized wedges
2–3 tablespoons olive oil
1 teaspoon paprika
Pinch of cayenne pepper or chilli powder (optional)
Salt

When I was growing up, I was an incredibly fussy eater with a very restricted diet that consisted mostly of cheese, chocolate, spaghetti bolognese and chilli con carne. This 'healthified' version of chilli non-carne is utterly delicious, and so much better for you. I love offsetting it with the fresh taste of the guacamole. If you want to go all out and make a Mexican feast, then I've included a wonderful recipe for spicy baked potato wedges. I love to dip them in the chilli – they absorb all the flavour and taste incredible. They're totally optional, but so yummy, and great for you too. You could otherwise serve this with brown rice, lemon-infused quinoa (see page 126), gluten-free tortilla chips or toasted gluten-free tortillas.

Start by preheating the oven to 190°C/170°C fan/gas 5. If you're making the potato wedges, add them to a roasting tin, then drizzle with the olive oil and add the paprika and cayenne or chilli powder and a big pinch of salt. Mix with your hands to ensure the potatoes are well coated, then place in the oven, on the top shelf, to cook for around 50 minutes, until deliciously soft in the middle and crunchy on the outside.

Just after you've put the potatoes in the oven, place the sweet potatoes in a roasting tin, drizzle with the olive oil add a pinch of salt and pop in the oven, on the middle shelf, to roast for around 30 minutes or until tender.

Recipe continues overleaf

Guacamole

4 avocados, peeled
   and stoned
12 cherry tomatoes, halved
1 red onion, peeled and
   finely chopped
1 big handful of fresh
   coriander, finely chopped
Juice of 2 limes
Pinch of salt

TIP

If your spice rack is lacking,
no worries – as long as you've
got the red chilli in the dish,
it will still have lots of flavour.

Recipe continued

To make the chilli, first add the onion, red peppers and crushed garlic to a pan and sauté over a medium-high heat for around 5 minutes, before adding the chilli, spices and ¼ teaspoon salt and cooking for a further 5 minutes.

Add the kidney beans and chopped tomatoes to the pan. Bring to the boil, then reduce the heat and simmer for 25 minutes, stirring frequently to make sure nothing sticks to the bottom of the pan. Just before you're done, add the roasted sweet potatoes and mix in well before cooking for a further 1–2 minutes.

To make the guacamole, simply mash the avocado flesh in a bowl until smooth, then add the remaining ingredients and stir until fully combined. Sprinkle the coriander over the chilli and serve with the guacamole and spicy potato wedges (if using). Delicious!

SWITCH IT UP

If you're not a big fan of sweet potato (apologies – it's used a lot in this book!), then use butternut squash, carrots or regular potatoes instead.

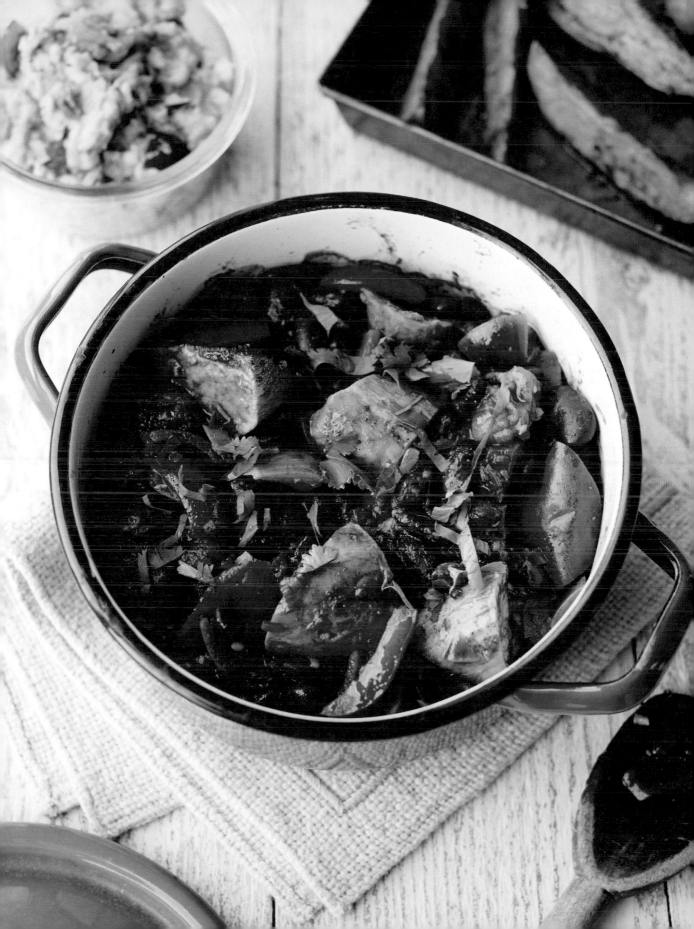

Vegan enchiladas

SERVES 2–3

6 gluten-free tortilla wraps

Spicy sweet potato and tomato filling
2–3 tablespoons olive oil
1 red onion, peeled and finely chopped
2 medium-sized sweet potatoes, peeled and cut into thumbnail-sized pieces
150g (1½ cups) sliced white mushrooms
1 teaspoon deseeded and finely chopped red chilli (or to taste)
120ml (½ cup) passata
1 x 180g bag of spinach

Avocado cream
2 avocados, peeled and stoned
Juice of 2 limes
2 tablespoons extra-virgin olive oil
Pinch of salt

TIP

Make sure to taste the chilli to see how spicy it is before you cook with it. You don't want an enchilada that's going to make your eyes water!

As you can see from the recipes in this chapter, Mexican-style dishes feature large. I've always loved the cuisine from that part of the world – the fresh, palate-tingling flavours and vibrant colours. This recipe is a really fun one to make and eat, too – I'm constantly preparing it for family lunches or casual dinners with friends.

Preheat the oven to 180°C/160°C fan/ gas 4. Heat the olive oil in a pan and add the onion, sweet potatoes, mushrooms and chilli, then sauté over a medium heat for 10–15 minutes, stirring regularly, until everything is well cooked. Add the passata and spinach, and cook until the spinach has completely wilted.

Spread your tortilla wraps out and place 3 generous spoonfuls of the mixture along the middle of each tortilla, then roll each one up and place in a baking dish. Put in the oven and bake for 20–25 minutes until golden brown and piping hot.

While the enchiladas are cooking, make the avocado cream by whizzing all the ingredients in a blender until smooth. Alternatively, you can simply mash the avocados with the other ingredients until smooth.

Take the enchiladas out of the oven when they're done and pour the avocado cream over the dish. Serve at once and enjoy!

GREEDY FOR GOODNESS?
Instead of regular salt, bleached to make it white, use pink Himalayan salt. Rich in vitamins and minerals, this is the purest form of salt you can get, as close to its natural state as possible.

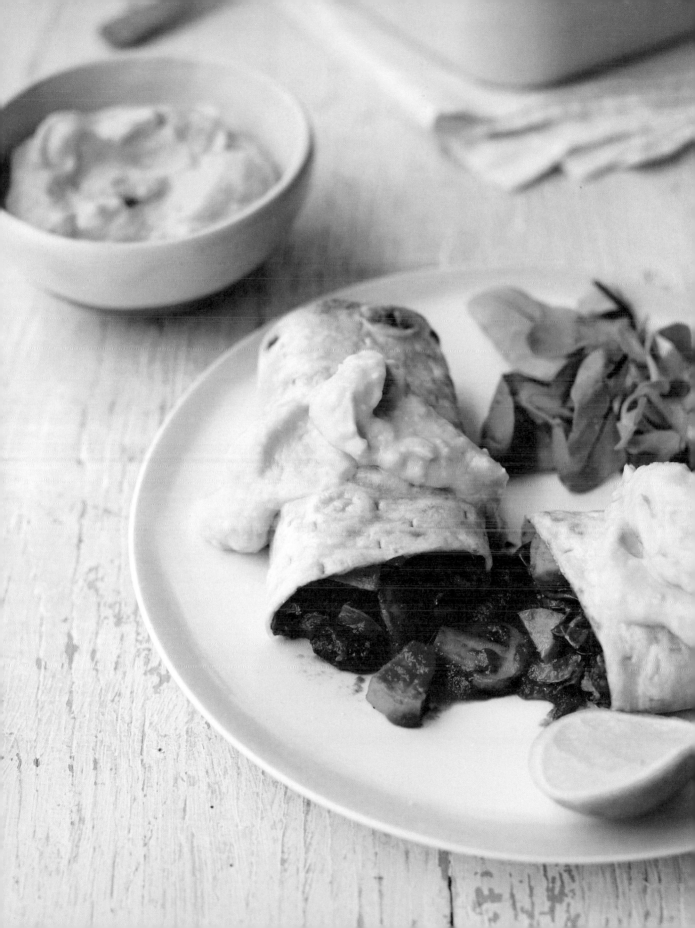

Turmeric-roasted cauliflower, garlic rice and tahini-cumin sauce

45 minutes or less

SERVES 2

120g (⅔ cup) brown rice
300ml (1¼ cups) boiling
    water
Juice of 1 lemon
2 tablespoons tamari
Salt and pepper

**Turmeric-roasted
cauliflower**
1 cauliflower (about 500g),
    trimmed and cut
    into florets
1 red onion, peeled
    and chopped
1 x 400g tin of chickpeas
1 clove of garlic, peeled
    and finely chopped
2 tablespoons olive oil
1 tablespoon turmeric

Tahini-cumin sauce
2 tablespoons tahini
Juice of 1 lemon
2 tablespoons hot water
½ teaspoon ground cumin

TIP

A powerful anti-
inflammatory, turmeric
is most effective when you
add a little black pepper –
this aids the absorption
and assimilation of the
nutrients in your body.

This dish was inspired by a meal two of my
flatmates were eating one evening in front of the
TV – what looked like a microwaved dish of yellow
cauliflower and white rice. It wasn't the look of the
dish that inspired me, but the wonderful spicy smell.
The turmeric-roasted cauliflower, caramelised
onions and garlic-infused rice go so well together,
while the tahini-cumin sauce adds a real depth of
flavour. Needless to say, the microwaved ready
meal has now been replaced!

Pour the rice into a saucepan with the water and
a pinch of salt and bring back up to the boil. Reduce
the heat, cover with a lid and simmer for around
40 minutes or until the rice is fluffy and tender
and the liquid fully absorbed.

Meanwhile, preheat the oven to 190°C/170°C fan/gas
5. Put the cauliflower, red onion, chickpeas and garlic
into a roasting tin. Drizzle over the olive oil, sprinkle
in the turmeric, ¼ teaspoon salt and a little pepper,
and mix together well to ensure the cauliflower and
chickpeas are really well coated in the spice mixture.
Place in the oven to roast for around 25 minutes,
tossing once or twice, until the cauliflower is tender
and lightly browned at the edges.

Make the tahini-cumin sauce by simply combining
all the ingredients in a bowl and mixing until smooth.
When the rice is cooked, stir in the lemon juice and
tamari. Spread the rice in the bottom of a wide serving
dish, topping with the turmeric-roasted cauliflower
and generously drizzling with the tahini-cumin sauce.

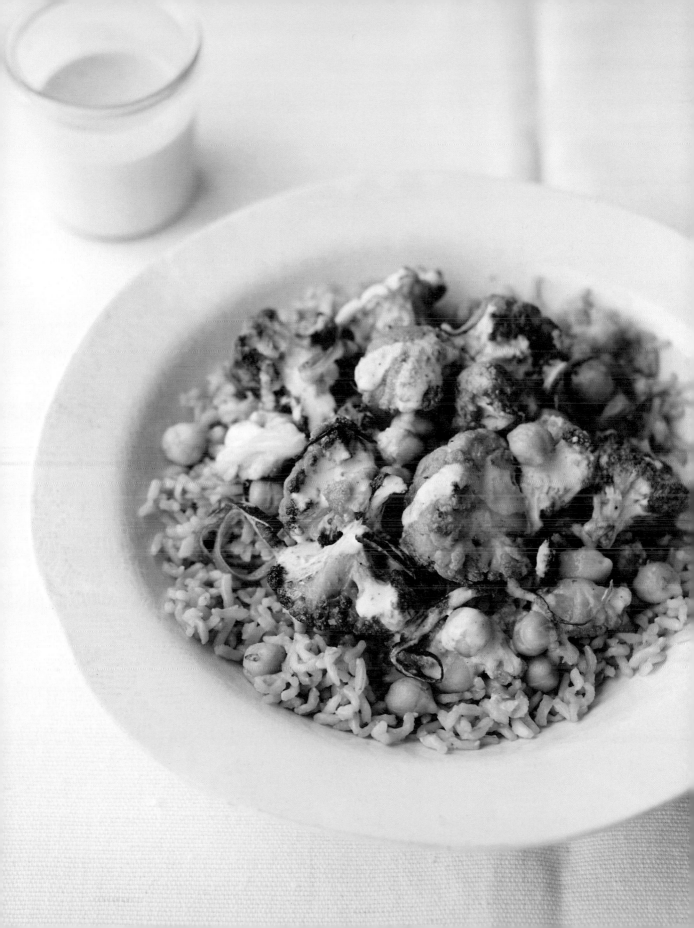

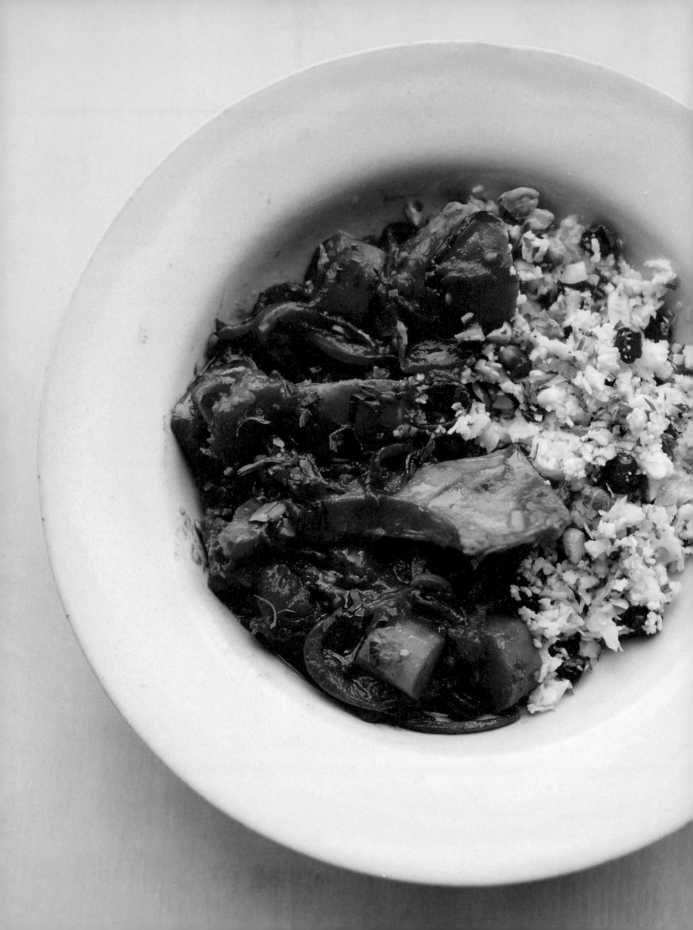

Moroccan root tagine and cauliflower couscous

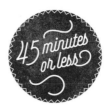

SERVES 4

Moroccan root tagine
2 medium-sized sweet
    potatoes, peeled and
    cut into small cubes
2 carrots, peeled and
    cut into small chunks
1 medium-sized butternut
    squash, peeled, deseeded
    and cut into small cubes
2 tablespoons olive oil
Salt

Tomato sauce
1–2 tablespoons olive oil
1 large red onion, peeled
    and chopped
2 cloves of garlic, peeled
    and finely chopped
1 teaspoon peeled and finely
    chopped fresh root ginger
1 tablespoon turmeric
2 teaspoons ground
    cinnamon
3 Medjool dates, pitted
    and chopped
2 x 400g tins of chopped
    tomatoes

Cauliflower couscous
80g (⅓ cup) raw pistachio
    kernels
1 large cauliflower, trimmed
    and cut into florets
Seeds from ½ pomegranate
Juice of 1 lemon
Sprig of parsley, finely
    chopped, plus extra
    to garnish

Moroccan cuisine is famous for its glorious spices and warming tagines. This recipe is both gently spiced and incredibly warming – a dish I'll never grow tired of. The 'couscous' is actually made from cauliflower, which may seem a little bizarre, but works remarkably well, providing a delicious gluten- and grain-free alternative.

Preheat the oven to 190°C/170°C fan/gas 5. For the tagine, place the root vegetables and squash into a roasting tin, drizzle over the olive oil and add a pinch of salt. Pop in the oven to roast for around 30 minutes or until the vegetables are tender.

Spread the pistachios for the cauliflower couscous on a baking tray, place in the oven and toast for around 7 minutes, shaking the pan from time to time to ensure they don't burn, then remove from the oven and set aside.

Meanwhile, make the tomato sauce. Add the olive oil to a pan, followed by the onion, garlic and ginger, and fry over a medium-high heat for 2 minutes. Add the spices, dates, tinned tomatoes and a generous pinch of salt and bring to the boil. Reduce to a slightly lower heat and cook for a further 2–3 minutes, then remove from the heat and set aside.

Next place the cauliflower florets into a blender or food processor and pulse until the consistency of

Recipe continues overleaf

The smaller the pieces of root vegetables and squash, the more quickly they'll roast. Chop chop!

Recipe continued

couscous or rice. (Alternatively, you can use a grater to grate the cauliflower.)

Transfer the 'couscous' to a bowl. If you wish to eat it raw, now is the time to add all the other ingredients, plus a pinch of salt. If you would prefer to heat it, add 1 tablespoon olive oil to a pan and sauté the cauliflower in the lemon juice before mixing in the other ingredients.

Once the root vegetables and squash have finished cooking, remove from the oven and add to the tomato sauce in the pan, heating through for 5 minutes until piping hot. Serve with the cauliflower couscous, garnished with fresh parsley.

SWITCH IT UP

Cauliflower couscous doesn't appeal? Or you simply can't be bothered to grate it? That's absolutely fine – we all have those days! Why not try using quinoa in its place? This recipe serves 4, so you'll need 250g (1½ cups) quinoa – boil in 700ml (3 cups) lightly salted water for 15–20 minutes or until fluffy before mixing with the other ingredients.

Sweet potato and spinach dhal with chickpea naan bread

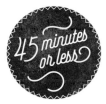
45 minutes or less

SERVES 2

Sweet potato and spinach dhal
1 large sweet potato, peeled and cut into small cubes
1 medium-sized red onion, peeled and finely chopped
1 teaspoon deseeded and finely chopped red chilli (or to taste)
100g (½ cup) dried red split lentils
475ml (2 cups) vegetable stock (made with a stock cube or bouillon powder)
1 teaspoon turmeric
1 teaspoon garam masala
1 x 180g bag of spinach

Chickpea naan bread
45g (½ cup) chickpea flour (besan or gram flour)
160ml (⅔ cup) water
Pinch of salt
2 tablespoons olive oil, for frying

To garnish (optional)
1 teaspoon black mustard seeds
2 tablespoons diced tomato
2 tablespoons diced cucumber
2 tablespoons chopped coriander

TIP

Test your chilli before using it. Better to burn your mouth before, than everyone else's afterwards!

Back when I was growing up, Friday nights meant a big Indian takeaway. I was always a fan of the Creamy Korma or the Spinach Dhal – two very different dishes, but the only ones I would ever order. Since then, while my diet has changed radically, the type of meals I crave have not. This Sweet Potato and Spinach Dhal is even more delicious than the ones I obsessed over years ago, and the most ironic part – it's quicker than ordering and waiting for your delivery, and a lot cheaper too! While the naan bread I've included here is by no means as light and fluffy as standard naan bread, it's a really awesome alternative and goes so well with the texture of the dhal.

In a large pan, combine all the ingredients for the dhal, except the spinach. Bring to the boil, then reduce the heat and simmer for 20–25 minutes until the sweet potato and lentils are tender. Just before the dhal is done, add the spinach and cook for a minute or two until wilted.

Meanwhile, make the naan bread. Combine all the ingredients in a mixing bowl and beat well until the batter is smooth. Heat a cast-iron or heavy-based frying pan, about 22cm in diameter, over a medium heat and add half the olive oil to the pan.

When the oil is hot, pour half the batter into the pan, spreading it around in a thin, even layer. Cook for 3–4

Recipe continues overleaf

Recipe continued

minutes on the first side, then flip over with a spatula and cook for a further minute or two on the other side. Repeat with with remaining batter to make the second naan. Your frying pan may get very hot during cooking. If the batter is over-bubbling when you pour it into the pan, reduce the heat slightly or even turn it off briefly. You want your bread to be able to able to cook for a few minutes without burning.

When the dhal is cooked, divide between bowls and garnish, if you like, with a sprinkling of mustard seeds, diced tomato, cucumber and coriander. Serve each bowl with a naan on the side.

SWITCH IT UP

Sweet potato and butternut squash are pretty interchangeable here, so do switch one for the other; likewise kale for the spinach.

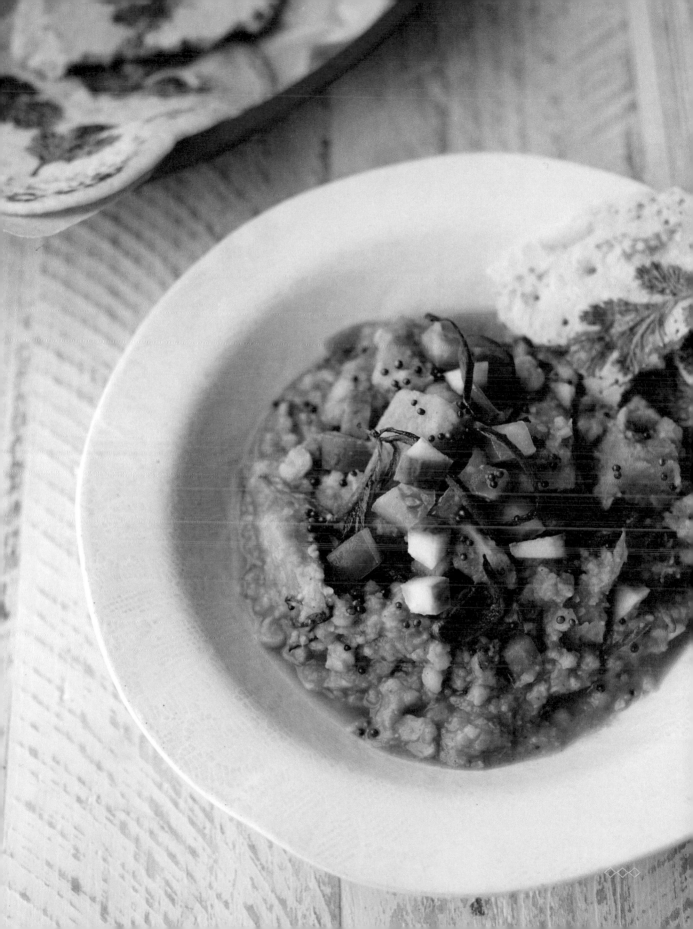

Spicy squash and black bean burgers

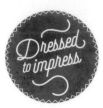

MAKES 8 BURGERS

½ medium-sized butternut
squash, peeled, deseeded
and cut into small cubes
5 tablespoons olive oil
1 x 400g tin of black beans,
drained and rinsed
1 red onion, peeled and diced
70g (½ cup) tinned
sweetcorn
2 teaspoons ground cumin
1 teaspoon chilli powder
2 teaspoons ground oregano
100g (1 cup) (gluten-free)
rolled oats, ground briefly
in a food processor to
breadcrumb consistency
Salt

Tahini sauce
4 tablespoons tahini
2 tablespoons extra-virgin
olive oil
2 tablespoons tamari
Juice of 2 limes

To serve
8 cos lettuce leaves
Hummus (to make your
own, see page 165)
Slices of avocado

TIP

If your mixture is still too
sticky to shape into burgers,
you may have ground the oats
too finely. Add extra ground
oats until you reach the
right consistency.

These burgers are amazing. The texture is to die for, and with a bit of crunch from the lettuce, this makes the perfect summer meal.

Preheat the oven to 190°C/170°C fan/gas 5. Place the squash in a roasting tin, drizzle with 2 tablespoons of the olive oil, add a pinch of salt and cook for around 30 minutes, turning occasionally, until tender. Meanwhile, place the beans in a large mixing bowl and, using a potato masher, mash until roughly half the mixture becomes a paste. Put to one side.

Add 1 tablespoon of the olive oil to a frying pan, followed by the onion, and cook over a medium-high heat for 5–7 minutes until caramelised. Add to the beans in the bowl, along with the sweetcorn, spices, oregano and ¼ teaspoon salt.

Once the squash is cooked, remove from the oven (leaving it switched on) and mash well before adding to the other ingredients in the bowl. Mix well and then add the ground oats to bind the mixture. Shape into 8 large patties 2–3cm thick and place in the fridge to set.

To cook, heat the remaining olive oil in a frying pan and fry the burgers for 3 minutes on each side, cooking them in two batches. Place on a baking tray and cook in the oven for 10–15 minutes or until crisp.

While the burgers are baking, make the tahini sauce. Mix all the ingredients together until smooth and heat up in a saucepan until piping hot. Serve each burger in a lettuce leaf with hummus, slices of avocado and a big drizzle of tahini sauce.

SWITCH IT UP

You can change the butternut squash for sweet potato, and ground oats for almond meal or brown rice flour. As long as everything is in the same quantities, it's smooth sailing.

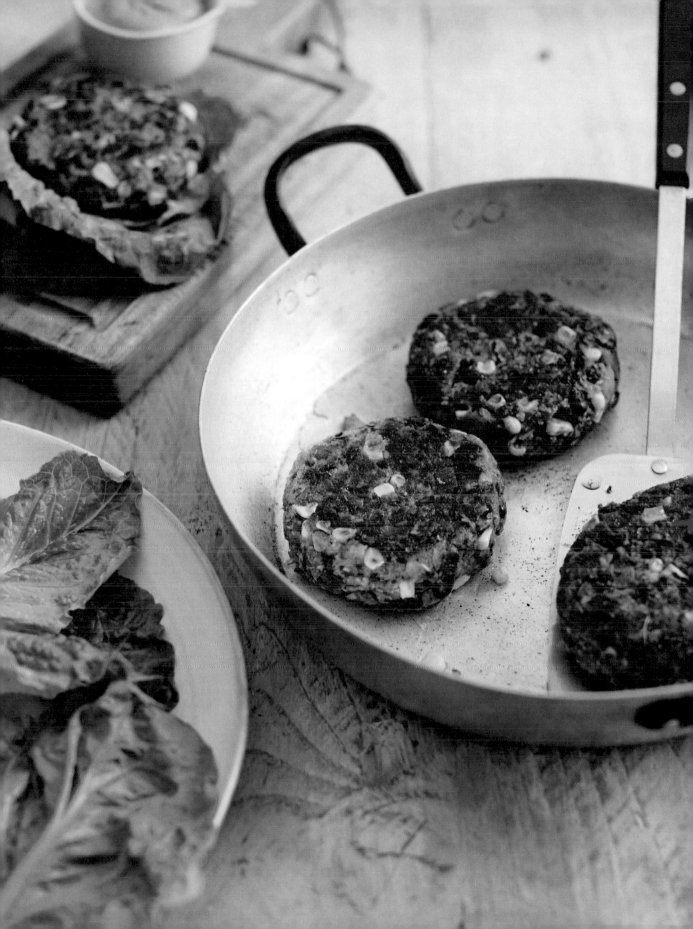

Quinoa with orange-chilli kale and roasted butternut squash

SERVES 2

1 medium-sized butternut
   squash, peeled, deseeded
   and cut into small cubes
4 tablespoons olive oil
85g (½ cup) quinoa
240ml (1 cup) boiling water
Juice of 1 lemon
½ clove of garlic, peeled
   and crushed
1–2 teaspoons deseeded
   and finely chopped red
   chilli (to taste)
300g kale, stems removed
   and leaves finely chopped
4 tablespoons freshly
   squeezed orange juice
2 tablespoons tamari
Salt

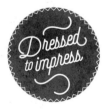

I love kale – in salads, smoothies or made into crisps (see page 168) – but I'd give them all up for this! Here the kale is wilted, then seasoned with garlic, chilli, orange and tamari, which has to be one of my favourite combos. The warmth, spice and sweetness all shine through. I'm pretty sure that a single forkful would turn any kale hater into a kale lover.

◇◇◇◇◇◇◇◇◇◇◇◇◇◇◇◇◇◇◇◇◇◇◇◇◇◇◇◇◇◇◇◇◇◇

Preheat the oven to 190°C/170°C fan/gas 5. Put the butternut squash in a roasting tin, drizzle over half the olive oil, add a pinch of salt and place in the oven to cook for around 30 minutes, checking every so often and giving it a stir to ensure it doesn't burn.

Meanwhile, add the quinoa to a saucepan with the water and a pinch of salt. Bring back up to the boil, then reduce to a simmer and cook for 15–20 minutes or until fluffy. Mix the lemon juice into the quinoa just before serving.

Now add the remaining olive oil to a frying pan and toast the chilli and garlic over a medium-high heat for 2–3 minutes or until fragrant, then add the kale and stir-fry until it starts to wilt. Finally, add the orange juice and tamari and cook for a further minute or two.

To assemble, first spread the quinoa on each plate or bowl, followed by the kale and then the caramelised butternut squash.

SWITCH IT UP

Also try serving this with crushed roasted walnuts, pine nuts or pecans.

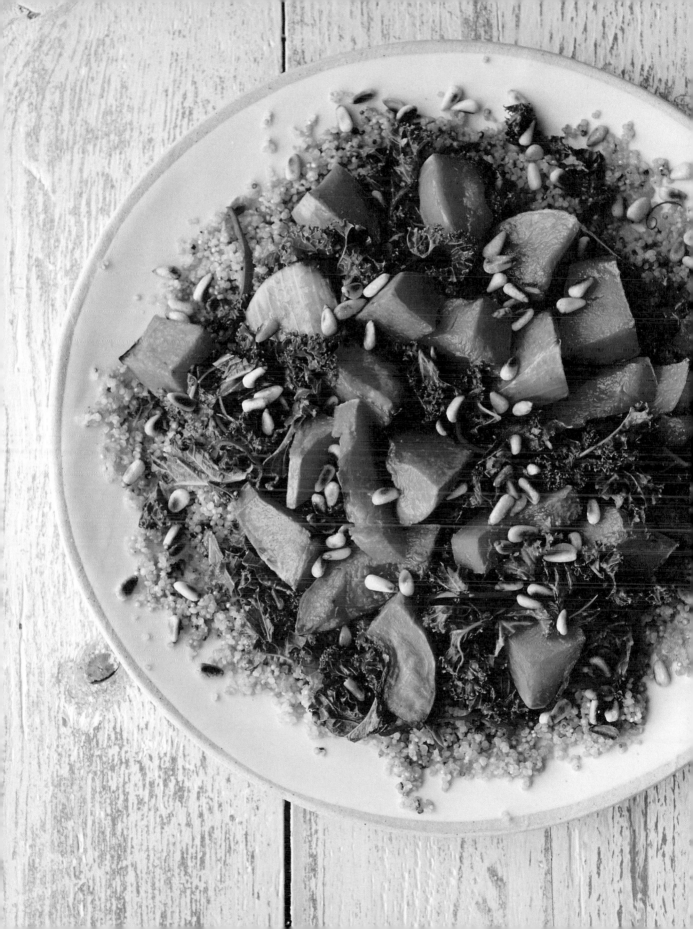

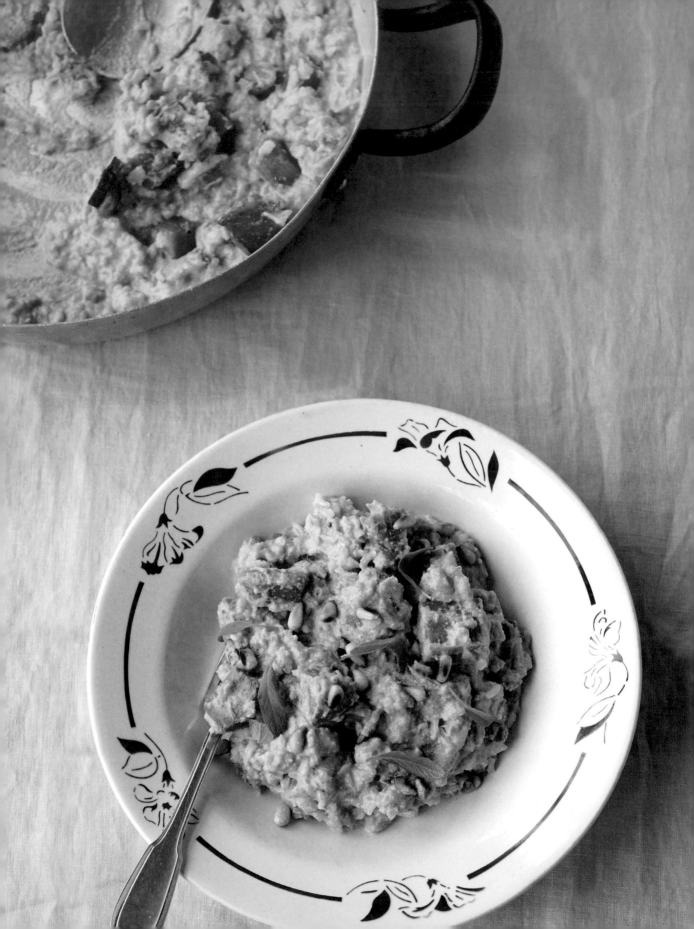

Creamy butternut squash and sage risotto

SERVES 3–4

150g (¾ cup) brown rice
475ml (2 cups) hot vegetable
stock (made with a stock
cube or bouillon powder),
plus extra if needed

Butternut squash cream
1 medium-sized butternut
squash, peeled, deseeded
and cubed
1 medium-sized red onion,
peeled and chopped
1–2 tablespoons olive oil
Pinch of salt
120g (1 cup) raw cashews,
soaked in water for at
least 2 hours or overnight,
then drained
4 tablespoons nutritional
yeast
120–240ml (½–1 cup)
water (start with less
and add more)
1 big handful of fresh
sage, chopped

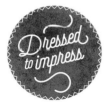

While I could describe every recipe in this book as 'my favourite recipe', I have to say that this particular dish, when made right, could knock the socks of any risotto! It's so creamy, filling, warming and nourishing, the creaminess coming from the butternut squash and cashew cream stirred into the brown rice. The balance of sweet and caramelised with salty is just right and I haven't met anyone who doesn't absolutely love this dish as much as I do.

◇◇◇◇◇◇◇◇◇◇◇◇◇◇◇◇◇◇◇◇◇◇◇◇◇◇◇◇◇◇◇◇◇◇◇◇◇◇

Preheat the oven to 190°C/170°C fan/gas 5. Place the butternut squash and onion in a roasting tin. Drizzle over the oil, add the salt and pop in the oven, tossing once or twice, to roast for 30 minutes or until tender.

Meanwhile, add the rice to a pan with the stock. Bring back up to the boil, then lower the heat and leave to simmer for around 40 minutes, topping up with extra stock or water if needed. Fully cooked, the rice should be soft and fluffy.

When the sweet potato are onion are cooked, remove from the oven and place half in a high-powered blender or a food processor with all the other ingredients for the cream. Blend until smooth, adding more water if needed.

When the rice is cooked, mix in the butternut squash cream and stir in the extra roasted squash and the sage. Plate up and enjoy!

GREEDY FOR GOODNESS?
If you want to get your 'green' fix for the day, this dish goes really well with some wilted spinach. Stir 180g into the creamy risotto at the final stage.

Ratatouille pasta with Brazil nut Parmesan

SERVES 4

220g (2 cups) dried brown
    rice fusilli or penne

Ratatouille
2 large aubergines,
    cut into small cubes
1 medium-sized butternut
    squash, peeled, deseeded
    and cut into small cubes
4 courgettes, sliced into
    circles
2 red peppers, deseeded
    and cut into chunks
24 cherry tomatoes, halved
1 red onion, peeled and sliced
2 cloves of garlic, peeled
    and crushed
2 tablespoons olive oil
240ml (1 cup) passata
1 bunch of basil, chopped
Salt and pepper

Brazil nut Parmesan
125g (1 cup) Brazil nuts
2 tablespoons nutritional
    yeast
½ tsp salt
1 tablespoon fresh
    lemon juice

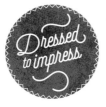

I love ratatouille – the flavours and textures of the different vegetables lend themself so well to a thick tomato sauce. The Brazil nut Parmesan, for sprinkling over at the end, is optional. Cheese made from nuts? I know it sounds bonkers, but it works.

◇◇◇◇◇◇◇◇◇◇◇◇◇◇◇◇◇◇◇◇◇◇◇◇◇◇◇

Preheat the oven to 190°C/170°C fan/gas 5. Add all the prepared vegetables to a roasting tin with the onion and garlic. Drizzle with olive oil and season with a pinch of salt, then place in the oven to roast for 35–45 minutes or until caramelised and tender, tossing every now and then to ensure they don't burn.

Make the 'Parmesan' now, if using: Process the nuts in a food processor until they form a fine crumb. Add the nutritional yeast, salt and lemon juice, mixing in with your hands. Spread on a baking tray lined with baking parchment and bake for 15–25 minutes, shaking the tin regularly to ensure the mix doesn't burn. Remove from the oven and allow to cool.

Shortly before the vegetables are cooked, bring a saucepan of salted water to the boil, add your pasta and cook according to the instructions on the packet – this is normally around 10 minutes.

Once the vegetables are done, tip them into a saucepan over a high heat and add the passata and lots of salt and pepper. Bring to the boil, then reduce the heat and let it bubble for 2–3 minutes, adding the basil just before serving. Drain the pasta, put into individual bowls and top with the ratatouille and a sprinkling of Brazil nut Parmesan.

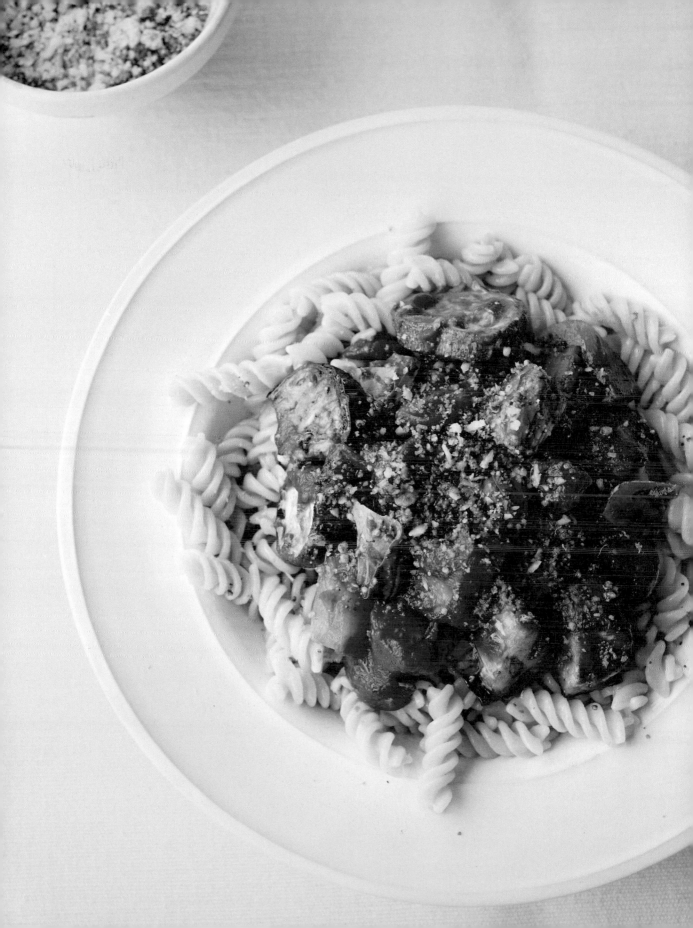

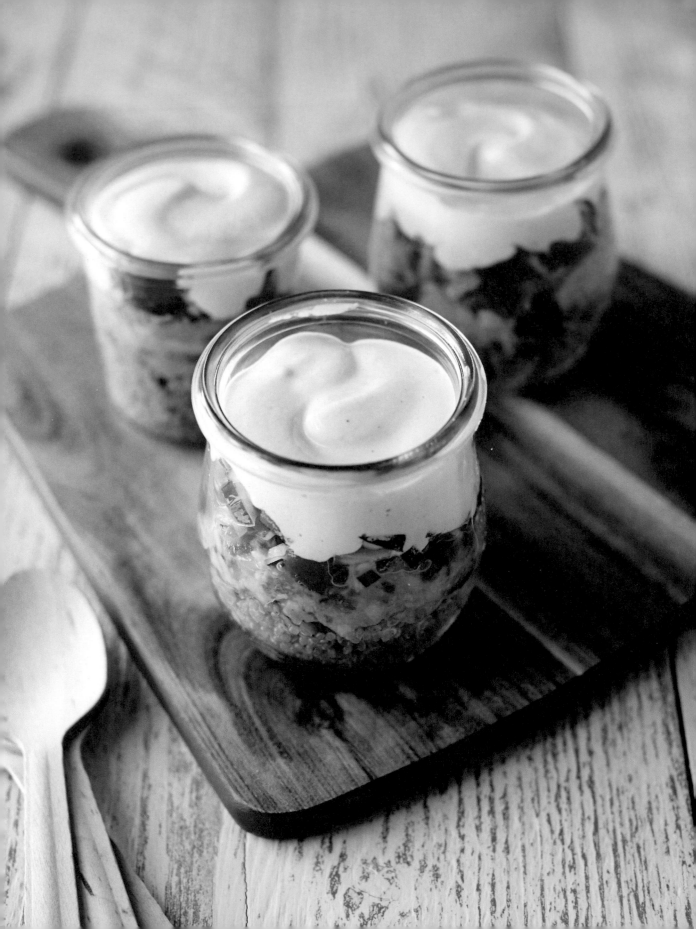

Mexican quinoa, guacamole and soured cream parfait

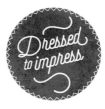

SERVES 4

85g (½ cup) quinoa
240ml (1 cup) boiling water
Juice of 1 lemon
Salt and pepper

Guacamole
1 large ripe tomato
2 ripe avocados, peeled
    and stoned
½ small red onion, peeled
    and finely chopped
1 red or green chilli, deseeded
    and finely chopped
Juice of 1 lime
1 handful of fresh coriander,
    finely chopped

Tomato salsa
12 cherry tomatoes,
    quartered
½ red onion, peeled
    and finely chopped
1 red pepper
2 tablespoons apple
    cider vinegar

Cashew soured cream
120g (1 cup) raw cashews,
    soaked in water for at
    least 2 hours or overnight,
    then drained
Juice of 1–2 lemons
2 teaspoons apple cider
    vinegar
120ml (½ cup) water

This savoury parfait has lots of layers, but don't let that put you off – they're each so simple to make! The base is a lemon-infused quinoa, topped with salsa, guacamole and cashew soured cream. An abundance of gorgeous textures and delicious, fresh flavours.

◇◇◇◇◇◇◇◇◇◇◇◇◇◇◇◇◇◇◇◇◇◇◇◇◇◇◇◇◇◇◇◇◇◇◇◇◇◇

Add the quinoa and water to a saucepan and bring back up to the boil, then reduce the heat and simmer for 15–20 minutes until light and fluffy, topping up with more water if needed. Remove from the heat and allow to cool before adding the lemon juice and a pinch of salt, mixing in well.

Meanwhile, make the guacamole. Use a large knife to pulverise the tomato to a pulp on your chopping bowl. Add to a bowl with the avocado flesh, then tip in the onion, chilli and lime juice and mash everything together into the texture you prefer. Add the coriander and mix in well, seasoning with salt and pepper to taste.

Combine all the ingredients for the tomato salsa in a small bowl, seasoning with salt and pepper to taste. Place all the ingredients for the cashew soured cream in a high-powered blender or a food processor and blend until smooth.

To assemble the layers of the parfait, simply add one at a time – the quinoa first, followed by the the guacamole, tomato salsa and finally the cashew soured cream. The parfait can be served in individual glasses/jars or one big glass bowl.

Lentil cottage pie with sweet potato mash

SERVES 4–6

6 large sweet potatoes,
   peeled and cut into chunks
80ml (⅓ cup) coconut cream
Generous pinch of salt
1–2 tablespoons olive oil
1 large red onion, peeled,
   halved and sliced
2 large carrots (500g in
   total), peeled and diced
1 red pepper, deseeded
   and diced
150g (1½ cups) sliced
   white mushrooms
2 tablespoons chopped
   thyme
350ml (1½ cups) vegetable
   stock (made with a stock
   cube or bouillon powder)
240ml (1 cup) passata
2 x 400g tins of green lentils,
   drained and rinsed

TIP

If you're assembling the
dish ahead and storing in
the fridge before cooking,
it'll need an extra 15 minutes
in the oven.

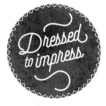

This is one of my favourite meals for a cosy night
in with friends or a family dinner party. The dish is
slow-cooked, but the pre-prep is an absolute doddle,
taking next to no time. I could eat this every day and
still crave more. The sweet potato mash is so thick
and indulgent. I've switched up the classic potato,
butter and cream mash to sweet potato and coconut
cream, making it a dish to remember.

◇◇◇◇◇◇◇◇◇◇◇◇◇◇◇◇◇◇◇◇◇◇◇◇◇◇◇◇◇◇

Preheat the oven to 190°C/170°C fan/gas 5. Next place
the sweet potatoes in a saucepan, cover with water and
boil for 15 minutes until tender. When cooked, drain
well and mash with the coconut cream. Season to taste
with some salt.

Meanwhile, place the olive oil in a frying pan, add the
red onion and fry over a medium-heat heat for 7–10
minutes until golden and caramelised. Now add the
carrots, red pepper, mushrooms and thyme and fry for
a further 5 minutes. Pour in the stock and the passata
and bring to the boil, then reduce the heat and simmer
for 10 minutes. Tip in the lentils, then cover with a lid
and simmer for another 10 minutes.

Pile the lentil mixture into a baking dish and spoon
the mash evenly on top. Place in the oven to cook
for 25 minutes until the sweet potatoes are nice
and crispy on top!

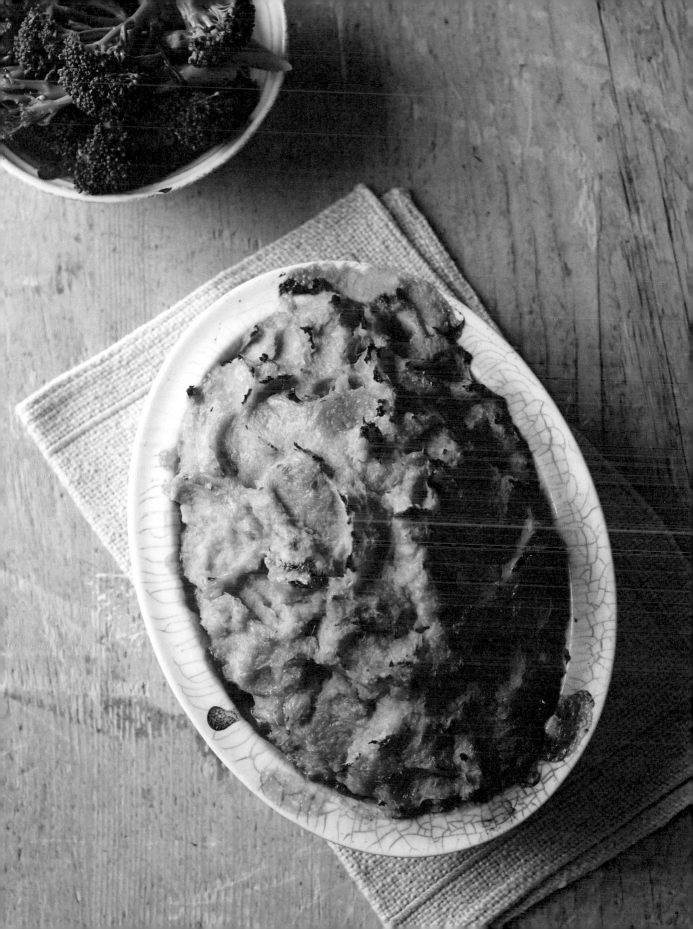

Brown rice pizza with a sun-dried tomato sauce

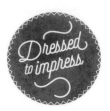

MAKES 1 PIZZA

Pizza base
220g (1¾ cups) brown
  rice flour
3 tablespoons arrowroot
½ tablespoon sea salt
½ teaspoon bicarbonate
  of soda
20g (⅓ cup) roughly
  chopped parsley
350ml (1½ cups) warm water
60ml (¼ cup) olive oil
1 tablespoon apple cider
  vinegar

Sun-dried tomato sauce
60g (1 cup) sun-dried
  tomatoes
2 tablespoons olive oil
60ml (¼ cup) passata
½ clove of garlic, peeled
  and crushed

Toppings
1 medium-sized squash,
  peeled, deseeded and
  cut into small cubes
1–2 tablespoons olive oil
Pinch of salt
150g (1½ cups) sliced
  white mushrooms
2 sweet peppers (any colour),
  deseeded and sliced
1 handful of fresh basil,
  roughly shredded
30g (¼ cup) pine nuts
50g (½ cup) pitted black
  olives
1 handful of rocket,
  to garnish

Who doesn't adore pizza?! This is a recipe I'm a little too obsessed with. I love playing around with the toppings and making single-sized portions for nights where comfort food is needed.

◇◇◇◇◇◇◇◇◇◇◇◇◇◇◇◇◇◇◇◇◇◇◇◇◇◇◇◇◇◇◇◇◇◇

Preheat the oven to 190°C/170°C fan/gas 5 and line a 30cm pizza tray or a baking sheet with baking parchment. Place the squash in a roasting tin, drizzle over the olive oil and add a pinch of salt. Pop in the oven to roast for 30 minutes or until tender.

Meanwhile, place all the ingredients for the pizza base in a mixing bowl and mix until fully combined. Scoop the dough out onto the prepared pizza tray/baking sheet and, with wet hands, flatten it out and mould into your pizza shape. You want a very thin crust, so it's best to spread the dough out as much as possible. Place in the oven and bake for 20 minutes until golden.

While the pizza base is cooking, place all the ingredients for the sun-dried tomato sauce into a blender and blend until smooth.

Remove the pizza from the oven and top with the sun-dried tomato sauce, mushrooms, peppers, basil, pine nuts and black olives. Cook for a further 10 minutes and serve, with the sweet potato cubes scattered on top and garnished with rocket leaves.

TIP

When making these for friends or family, it's always easier to make individual pizzas. People may like more or less of an ingredient and it also saves on all the slicing!

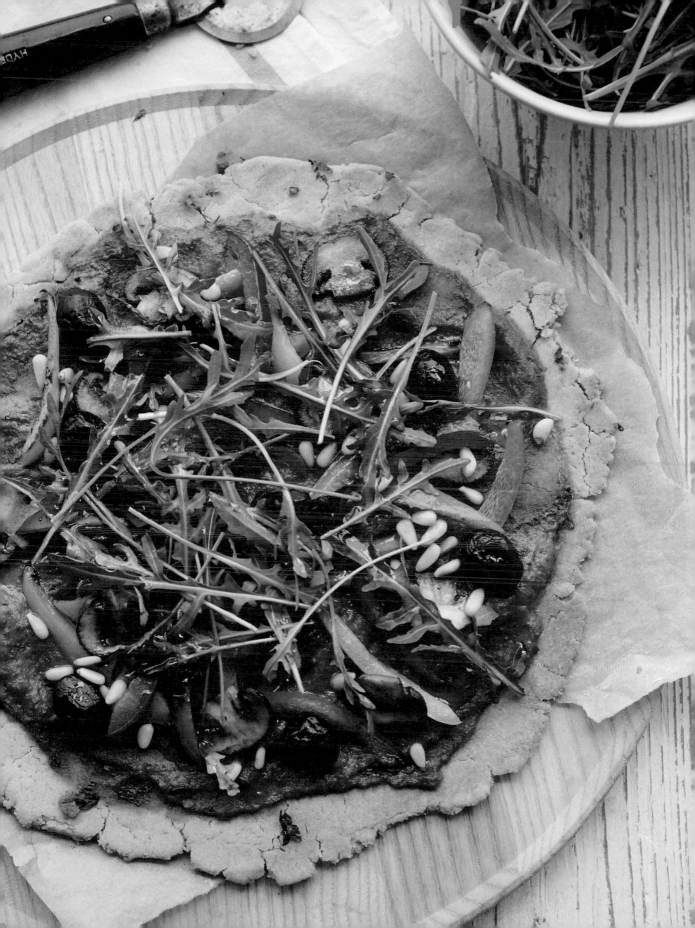

HOW TO MAKE A
Balance Bowl

The philosophy behind the balance bowl is a delicious, balanced meal that is incredibly straightforward to make and doesn't require any specific ingredients. You simply choose your favourites from the five categories below, or just use any leftovers you may have in the fridge. There are five categories: Grain, Main Vegetable, Extra Veggies, Protein and, most importantly, a kick-ass Dressing, for which I've given a selection of different sauces. While you can experiment and go wild with any of the first four categories, it's the dressing that's the most important – the component that truly makes (or breaks) the finished 'bowl'.

SERVES 1

GRAIN
Choose one of the following:
60g (⅓ cup) brown rice
60g (⅓ cup) quinoa
60g (⅓ cup) millet

Seasoning
Juice of ½ lemon
1 teaspoon tamari

MAIN VEGETABLE
Choose one of the following:
1 medium-sized butternut squash, peeled, deseeded and cut into small cubes
1 large sweet potato, peeled, deseeded and cut into small cubes
1 aubergine, cut into small cubes

To roast
2 tablespoons olive oil

EXTRA VEGGIES (OPTIONAL)
Choose as many or as few as you please from the following. (Cooking methods suggested in brackets if cooking from scratch)
2 large handfuls of spinach (steam or stir-fry)
2 large handfuls of kale, stems removed and leaves chopped (steam or stir-fry)
1 large carrot, peeled (cut into wedges and roast or chop thinly and stir-fry)
1 red pepper, deseeded and cut into chunks (roast)
12 cherry tomatoes, halved (roast or add to a stir-fry)
75g (½ cup) peas
100g white mushrooms (1 cup, halve and roast or slice and stir-fry)
1 courgette (cut into chunks and roast or slice and stir-fry)
1 beetroot, peeled (cut into wedges and roast or slice and stir-fry)
1 leek, chopped (stir-fry)
1 red onion, peeled (cut into wedges and roast or chop and stir-fry)

PROTEIN (OPTIONAL)
Choose as many/few as you please from the following:
130g (½ cup) tinned lentils
90–130g (⅓–½ cup) tinned beans
2 tablespoons seeds (sunflower, pumpkin, chia, sesame)
2 tablespoons nuts (cashews, almonds, pecans, brazil nuts, pine nuts)

DRESSING
Select one of the following:
Tomato, tamari, garlic and basil sauce
35g (⅓ cup) tinned chopped tomatoes
1 teaspoon tamari
1 good handful of fresh basil
¼ clove of garlic, peeled and crushed
Pinch of chilli powder (to spice things up a little – optional)

Garlic-tahini sauce

60g (¼ cup) light tahini
¼ clove of garlic, peeled and crushed
1–2 tbsp water (depending how thick
    or thin the tahini is)
Juice of ½ large lemon
1 teaspoon tamari
Pinch of salt

Citrus-tahini sauce

60g (¼ cup) light tahini
Juice of ⅓ lemon
Juice of 1 orange
1 tablespoon manuka honey or agave syrup
Salt and pepper to taste

Avocado and basil

1 avocado, peeled, stoned and sliced
Juice of 1 lemon
1 handful of fresh basil leaves, chopped
80ml (⅓ cup) water
Generous pinch of salt

Coconut and lemon sauce

80ml (⅓ cup) full-fat coconut milk
Juice of 1 lemon
1 teaspoon apple cider vinegar
Pinch of salt

'Cheesy' no cheese sauce

80ml (⅓ cup) full-fat coconut milk
2 heaped tablespoons nutritional yeast
80ml (⅓ cup) hot vegetable stock (made
    with a stock cube or bouillon powder)

Note
This sauce is perfect with cauliflower, for an
amazing cheese-less cauliflower cheese!

METHOD

Grain

First put your choice of grain on to boil – as
a rule of thumb, you want double the amount
of water to the grain, but do read the instructions
on the packet. When it's cooked, stir in the
lemon juice and tamari.

Main vegetable

Preheat the oven to 190°C/170°C fan/gas 5. Place
your choice of prepared vegetable in roasting tin,
add a drizzle of olive oil and place in the oven to
roast for 30 minutes or until soft.

Extra veggies

It's up to you how you cook any extra veggies –
indeed you could use up any cooked vegetables
you may have in the fridge. If cooking from
scratch, you can prepare as above and add some
(carrot, red pepper, tomatoes, mushrooms,
beetroot, red onion) to the roasting tin with the
main veg, sauté others (spinach, kale, carrot,
tomatoes, mushrooms, courgette, beetroot, leek,
red onion) in a frying pan for 5–10 minutes, or
even add others (spinach, kale, peas) to the pan
with the grains shortly before they have finished
boiling. Spinach, kale and peas can otherwise
be steamed for 3–4 minutes.

Protein

If you are adding protein, either mix in with the
grain (for the lentils or beans) or sprinkle on top
of the finished dish (nuts or seeds). To toast nuts
or seeds, place on a baking tray and cook with the
main vegetable in the oven for 5–7 minutes for
most nuts; around 4 minutes for seeds or pine
nuts. Check frequently, shaking the tray from
time to time, to ensure they don't burn. Remove
from the oven and allow to cool before chopping
up/crushing the nuts (if using) for sprinkling.

Dressing

Simply mix together all the ingredients for the
sauce of your choice. Some sauces can be heated
up, if you prefer. I tend to always heat up the
tomato, coconut and lemon and garlic-tahini
dressings, as well as the 'cheesy' sauce, before
adding them to the bowl.

Building your bowl

To make the bowl really appealing visually,
first add the cooked, seasoned grain, followed
by the vegetables and a good drizzle of the sauce/
dressing, sprinkling any toasted nuts or seeds
on top.

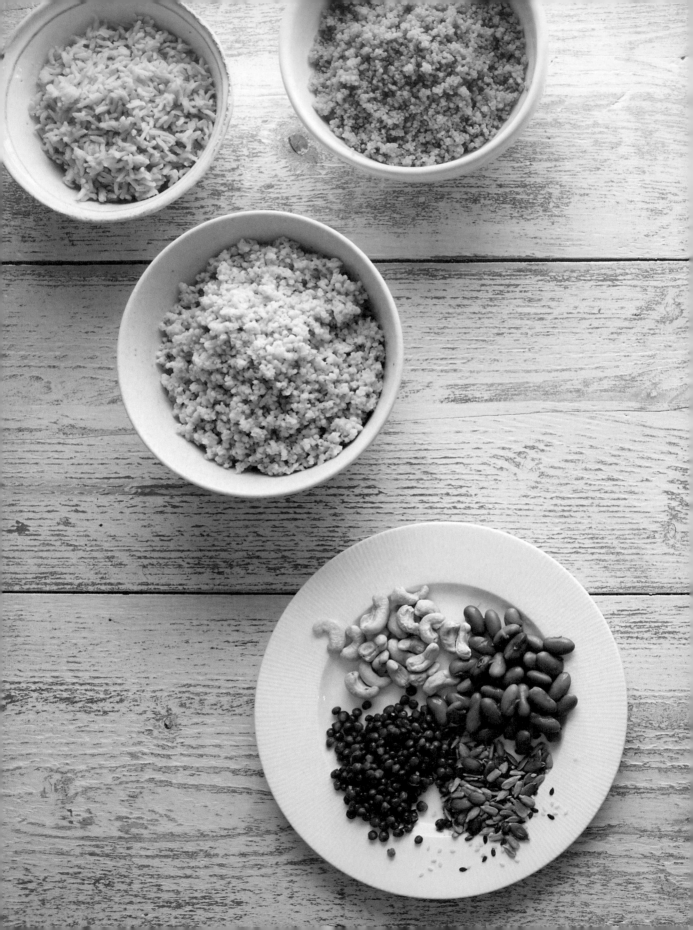

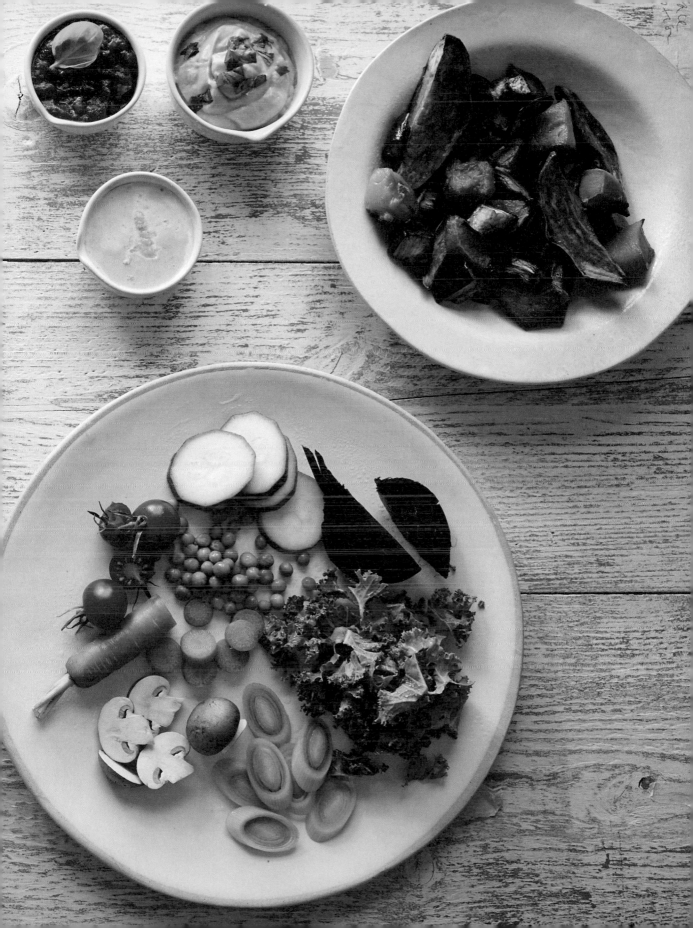

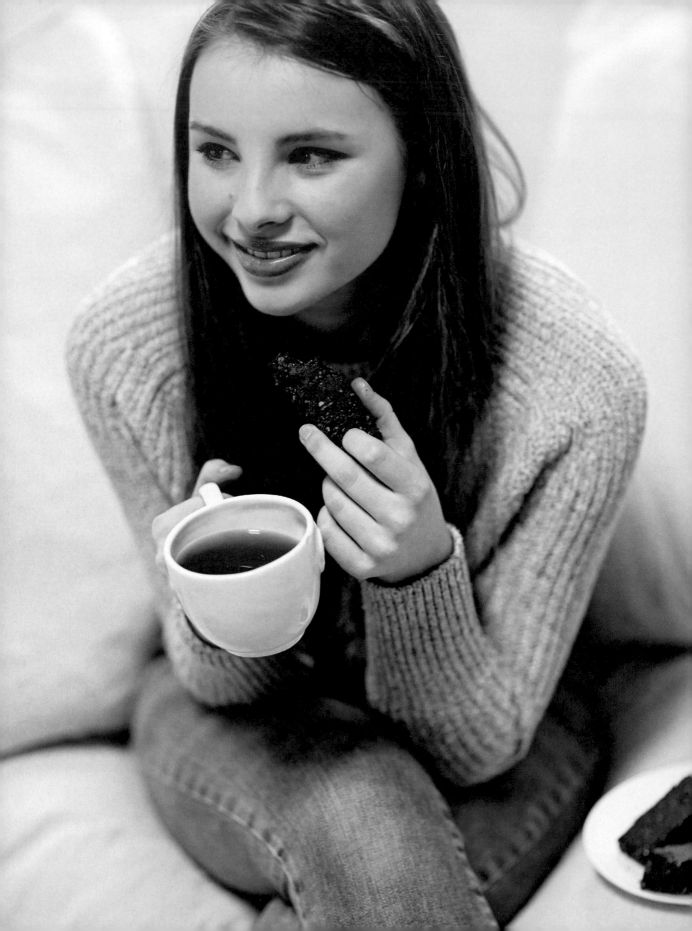

Snacking has to be one of my favourite things to do – not only because it gives an excuse to have a quick nibble of something delicious, but also because it breaks up the morning or afternoon and provides a burst of energy to keep you going.

It's these moments when you need to be prepared and have something tasty and nutritious to hand, as tracking down a healthy snack when you're out and about can be impossible. As with my lunches on the go (see previous chapter), a bit of forward thinking is the key – just 10 minutes at the weekend can mean effortless, healthy snacking for the week ahead. I'm a big fan of batch cooking, which does mean investing in a range of ingredients at the outset. You'll find you use them again and again, however, making them much more cost-effective in the long run and easier to prepare snacks on a whim.

This section is packed with my favourite sweet and savoury nibbles, simple recipes that will keep you fuelled during those 'hungry' moments between meals. From savoury goodies like my Kale crisps and Poppy seed crackers (see pages 168 and 169) to sweet treats like my flapjacks, Raw chocolate brownies and Peanut butter bites (see pages 174, 172 and 178), there are so many great options, all just as tasty (or even more so!) than their unhealthy counterparts. At the same time, they're all prepared with a proper balance of carbohydrates, protein and healthy fats that will work together to really support you through the day, giving your body the vital nutrients it needs.

Hummus

Basic hummus

I love having a big bowl of hummus to hand, and making your own is just so easy. All the equipment you need is a food processor and a finger to press 'blend' and, voilà, after a few minutes you've got a delicious, creamy bowl of hummus! I'm a hummus fanatic and end up adding it to most meals. A great source of protein and calcium, it makes a brilliant addition to your diet if you don't eat meat or dairy products.

MAKES 250G (2 CUPS) HUMMUS

1 x 400g tin of chickpeas,
    drained and rinsed
Juice of 1 lemon
1 tablespoon tahini
1 clove of garlic
2 tablespoons extra-virgin olive oil
1 teaspoon ground cumin
1 teaspoon paprika
Salt and pepper

Add the chickpeas to a food processor with all the other ingredients, then simply blend into a creamy purée, seasoning with salt and pepper to taste. Stored in an airtight container in the fridge, it will keep for around 5 days.

Sweet potato hummus

MAKES 250G (2 CUPS) HUMMUS

1 large sweet potato, peeled
    and cut into small cubes
4 tablespoons olive oil
Pinch of salt
1 x 400g tin of chickpeas,
    drained and rinsed
2 tablespoons almond butter
    or tahini (optional)
Juice of 1 lemon
1 teaspoon ground cumin
5 tablespoons water
2–4 tablespoons paprika

Preheat the oven to 200°C/180°C fan/ gas 6. Place the sweet potato cubes in a roasting tin, drizzle with half the olive oil, add the salt and roast in the oven for around 30 minutes. When they're crispy on the outside but still soft and gooey in the middle, then they're done! Remove from the oven and allow to cool slightly before mashing well.

Add all the other ingredients to a blender or food processor and blend into a smooth paste. (You may have to stop a few times to clean the blade as it can get quite sticky!) Add the mashed sweet potato to the blender/food processor and blend until combined and as smooth as you like!

(Both recipes photographed on pages 166–167)

Following page, clockwise from top left: Hummus, Root vegetable crisps, Sweet potato hummus, Gluten-free poppy seed crackers, Kale crisps.

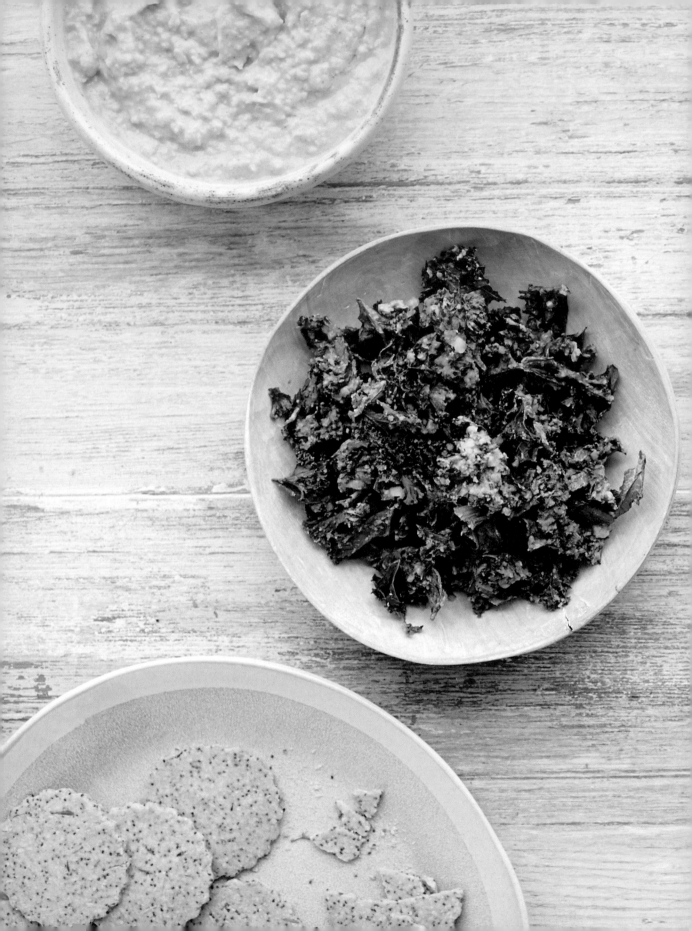

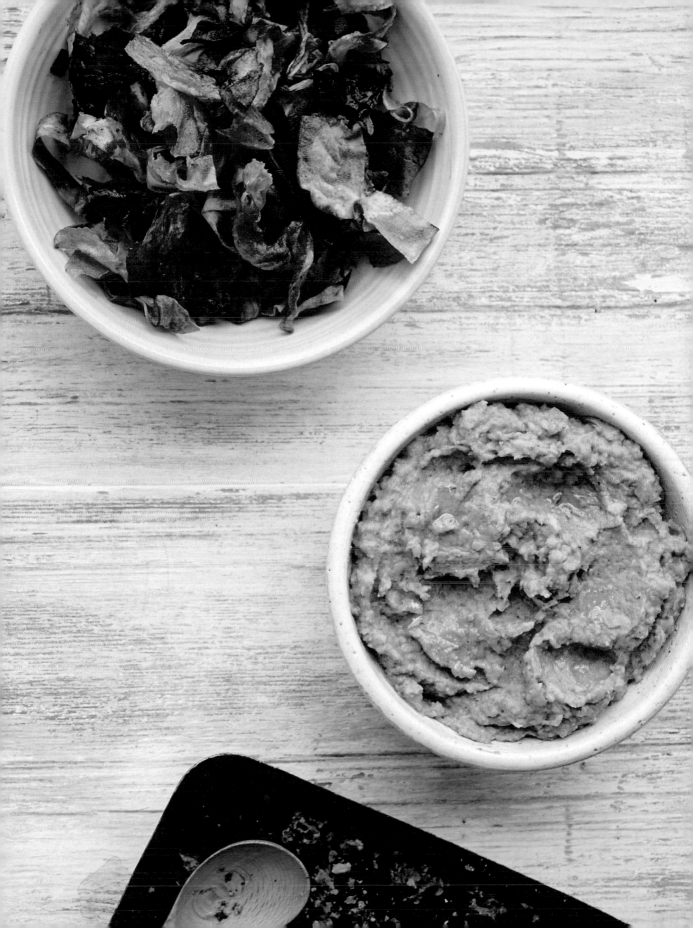

Kale crisps

SERVES 4–6

1 x 180g bag of kale

'Cheesy' seasoning
120g (1 cup) raw cashews, soaked in water for at least 2 hours or overnight, then drained
1 red pepper, deseeded and chopped
3 tablespoons lemon juice
2 tablespoons nutritional yeast

Kale crisps are irresistibly delicious, so much so that everyone in my family now makes them! You can buy kale crisps in supermarkets and cafés, but they really are pretty expensive for only a very small portion – which is why I always make mine at home. Call me greedy, or just sensible, but you definitely get more for your money and they actually taste better too! Not everyone has a fancy dehydrator for cooking crisps (in fact I'm pretty sure that most people don't!), so I've included instructions for cooking them in the oven too. (See photo on page 166).

◇◇◇◇◇◇◇◇◇◇◇◇◇◇◇◇◇◇◇◇◇◇◇◇◇◇◇

Preheat the oven (if using) to 120°C/100°C fan/gas ½ and line a baking tray with baking parchment. Rinse the kale and dry the leaves well, then remove the stems and tear the leaves into bite-sized pieces before placing in a large bowl.

Place all the ingredients for the 'cheesy' seasoning (it's all in the nutritional yeast!) in a high-powered blender or a food processor and blend until smooth.

Pour the mixture over the kale in the bowl and mix in well using your hands to ensure the leaves are completely coated. Spread the leaves out in the prepared baking tray and place in the oven to bake for around 30 minutes or until crispy.

Alternatively, spread the kale out on dehydrator trays and leave to dehydrate at 70°C for 10 hours, or until crunchy. Once made (by either method), the crisps can be stored in an airtight container or resealable plastic bag for up to 2 weeks.

Gluten-free poppy sced crackers

**MAKES ABOUT
24 CRACKERS**

60g (½ cup) brown rice flour,
   plus extra for dusting
85g (1 cup) ground almonds
¼ teaspoon bicarbonate
   of soda
2 tablespoons poppy seeds
½ teaspoon salt
½ teaspoon dried thyme
60ml (¼ cup) water
½ teaspoon olive oil

Coming up with the perfect gluten-free cracker was no easy task. I'm a fussy recipe creator and never settle for a recipe that's less than perfect. Sackfuls of almonds, flour and poppy seeds later, these crackers were finally born! The consistency and flavour are just as I'd hoped and I couldn't be happier with how easy they are to make. I love them dipped into big bowls of my Sweet potato hummus and guacamole. (See photo on page 166).

Preheat the oven to 180°C/160°C fan/gas 4 and line a baking tray with baking parchment. In a bowl, mix together the flour, almonds, bicarbonate of soda, poppy seeds, salt and thyme. Pour in the water and olive oil and mix well with a spoon before kneading the dough with your hands and shaping into a large ball.

Place the ball of dough on a piece of baking parchment and, with a floured rolling pin, roll the dough out until very thin. Use a 6cm fluted pastry cutter to stamp the dough into about 24 crackers. Pop on the baking tray and bake in the oven for around 20 minutes until golden.

Root vegetable crisps

1 large sweet potato
1 large beetroot
1 large parsnip
1 large carrot
½ teaspoon paprika
½ teaspoon salt
1 teaspoon coconut palm
    sugar (optional)
1 tablespoon extra-virgin
    olive oil

SWITCH IT UP

You can make these crisps
using just one root vegetable,
if you prefer, in the same
quantity as all four, or
follow this recipe to make
potato crisps!

I've always been much more of a sweet than
savoury girl, but one thing I can never resist are
these vegetable crisps. They're so simple to make,
and wonderfully satisfying to munch on. I always
make a big batch for when friends come over, dipped
into a big bowl of my Sweet Potato Hummus (see
page 165 for the recipe and page 167 for the photo).

Preheat the oven (if using) to 180°C/160°C fan/gas 4
and line a baking tray with baking parchment. Peel
all the vegetables and, using a mandolin or vegetable
peeler, thinly slice them before carefully placing
between layers of kitchen paper to absorb any
excess moisture.

Place the sliced vegetables in a bowl and add the
paprika, seasoning and olive oil. Toss well to make
sure every slice is coated in the oil mixture.

Spread out the vegetables in the prepared baking
tray and place in the oven to cook for 30 minutes,
checking every 10 minutes or so to make sure they're
not burning, tossing them in the tray, if necessary, to
cook on the other side. Remove from the oven and
leave them on the tray to cool and crisp up.

Alternatively, spread the vegetables out on dehydrator
trays and leave to dehydrate at 70°C for 10 hours,
or until crunchy. Once made (by either method),
the crisps can be stored in an airtight container or
resealable plastic bag for up to 10 days, though
they're best eaten within 4 days.

Trail mix

MAKES 1 BIG JAR

100g (2 cups) coconut flakes
120g (1 cup) raw cashews
115g (1 cup) pecans
140g (1 cup) pumpkin seeds
2 tablespoons coconut oil
2 tablespoons agave or
    pure maple syrup
1 teaspoon ground cinnamon
140g (1 cup) sultanas
55g (½ cup) dried goji berries

I think of the words 'trail mix' and I'm immediately taken back to when I was eight years old, setting off for school with a bag of nuts and raisins to snack on at break. They weren't all that delicious but relatively healthy, even so! This trail mix is super-easy to throw together and I'm forever making a jarful to sit in my pantry for when I get the munchies. It's so much yummier than any ready-made variety, as the nuts and seeds are roasted in a mixture of coconut oil, maple and cinnamon. Just a touch goes a long way and makes this a really tasty snack.

◇◇◇◇◇◇◇◇◇◇◇◇◇◇◇◇◇◇◇◇◇◇◇◇◇◇◇◇◇◇◇◇◇◇◇◇

Preheat the oven to 190°C/170°C fan/gas 5 and line a baking tray with baking parchment. Place the coconut flakes, cashews and pumpkin seeds in a bowl and mix together.

In a saucepan, melt the coconut oil and stir in the agave or maple syrup and the cinnamon. Pour the coconut mixture into the bowl with the dry ingredients and mix well to combine.

Spread the coated trail mix out on the prepared baking tray and pop in the oven to bake for 10–15 minutes. Check once or twice to make sure nothing burns, turning the mixture over in the tray with a spatula if it looks as though it's getting too brown.

Remove from the oven and leave to cool. Add the sultanas and goji berries and place in a clean jar, ready to take with you when you're on the go for when the munchies hit!

Bars and brownies

Raw gingerbread bars

When I was growing up, gingerbread was one of my favourite sweet treats. This raw version is even tastier, and so much better for you!

MAKES ABOUT 9 BARS

115g (1 cup) pecans
130g (1 cup) whole almonds
180g (1 cup) Medjool dates, pitted
1 tablespoon ground cinnamon
1 tablespoon ground ginger

Start by adding the pecans and almonds to a food processor, blending into a chunky crumb. Add the dates and spices and continue to process for 3–5 minutes until the mixture is really soft and dough-like.

Tip the mixture into an 18cm square baking tin, spreading it out and pressing it down into an even layer about 1cm thick. Place in the freezer for 30 minutes to set before slicing into 9 bars. Alternatively, you can pinch off sections of the dough and roll them into balls between your palms before placing in the freezer to set.

Raw chocolate brownie bars

This recipe is one that I almost regret creating – the brownies are just so delicious I end up devouring them in next to no time. But it's OK – they are amazing for you too! Made with pecans and Medjool dates, a protein-packed, energising combo, these brownies are a million times better for you than any shop-bought bar. I also love the fact they're made with only four ingredients – it just makes life so much simpler.

MAKES ABOUT 6 BARS

115g (1 cup) pecans
180g (1 cup) Medjool dates, pitted
2 tablespoons dried goji berries
55g (½ cup) raw cacao (or cocoa) powder

Place the pecans in a food processor and process into a fine crumb. Add the dates, goji berries and cacao powder and continue to blend until a dough-like ball forms.

Scoop up spoonfuls of the mixture and shape into roughly 6 bars each about 1cm thick. Store in an airtight plastic container in the fridge before serving. Kept like this, they'll last for up to 3 weeks.

SWITCH IT UP

Swap the pecans for almonds or cashews or, if you're allergic to nuts, to sunflower seeds.

Opposite, clockwise from top left: Sticky almond butter flapjacks, Raw gingerbread bars, Raw chocolate brownie bars.

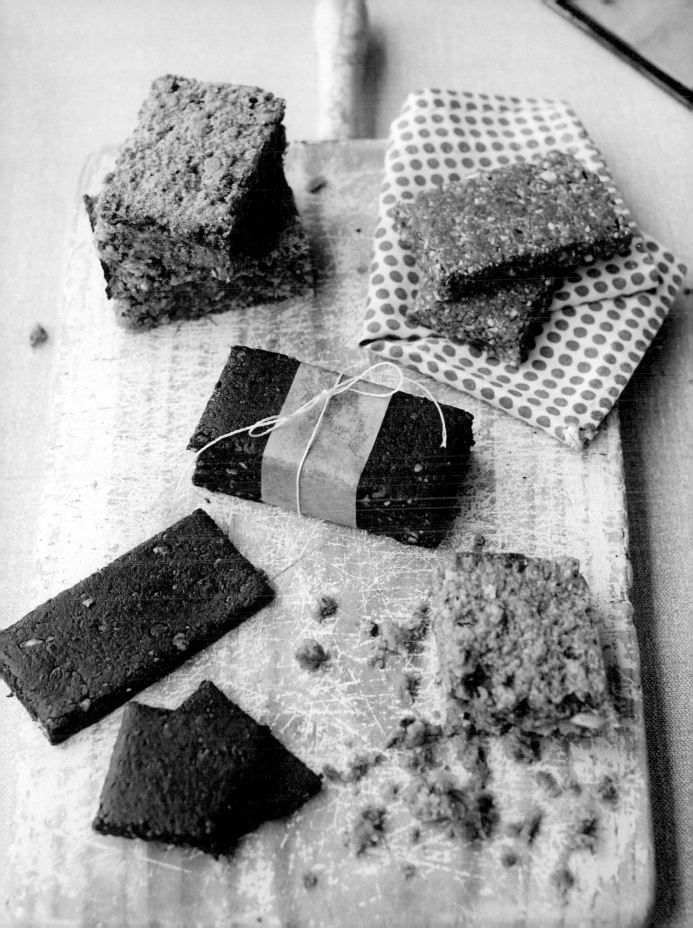

Sticky almond butter flapjacks

MAKES 12 FLAPJACKS

Coconut oil, for greasing
360g (2 cups) Medjool dates,
    pitted and chopped
475ml (2 cups) water
230g (1 cup) almond butter
300g (3 cups) (gluten-free)
    rolled oats
120g (1 cup) raw cashews
140g (1 cup) sunflower seeds

These flapjacks really are even tastier than the sugar-laden ones you buy from the supermarket. Something I've always disliked about flapjacks is how dry they can be, but these are sticky, gooey and so indulgent. Instead of refined sugars, I use a combination of dates and almond butter to sweeten the mixture and create that glorious stickiness!(See photo on page 173).

Preheat the oven to 160°C/140°C fan/gas 3, then grease a 25cm x 30cm baking tray with coconut oil and line with baking parchment. Place the dates and water in a saucepan, bring to the boil, then reduce the heat and simmer until soft. Tip the cooked dates into a food processor and blend into a smooth purée. Pour into a mixing bowl and add the almond butter.

Add all the remaining ingredients to the food processor and pulse until very finely chopped. You don't want it to turn into a flour, and yet you don't want it to be too crunchy – a happy medium!

Add the dry mix to the bowl with the date and almond butter mixture. With a wooden spoon, vigorously mix everything together until it's fully combined and every bit of the dry mix is coated in the date and almond butter.

Spoon into the prepared baking tray, spreading the mixture into an even layer 2–3cm deep. Place in the preheated oven and cook for around 20 minutes. Remove from the oven, cut into 12 bars and leave to cool down completely before removing from the tin.

Nut butter cups

**MAKES 6 NUT
BUTTER CUPS**

2 generous tablespoons
 coconut oil, melted
30g (¼ cup) raw cacao
 (cocoa) powder
3 tablespoons agave
 or pure maple syrup
6 teaspoons almond butter

Growing up, Reese's Peanut Butter Cups were my favourite snack. I could have eaten them for breakfast, lunch and dinner and I would still have been craving more! They were also the first thing that I tried to recreate when I started a sugar- and dairy-free diet, and once I mastered how to make them, there was no doubt in my mind that healthy eating was anything but boring! (See photo on page 176).

Add the melted coconut, cacao (or cocoa) powder and agave or maple syrup to a mixing bowl and mix until smooth. Add about 1 teaspoon of the liquid chocolate into the bottom of 6 cupcake cases – enough to cover the bottom of each paper case. Put in the freezer for 5 minutes or until the chocolate has hardened.

Remove from the freezer and add 1 teaspoon of almond butter to each chocolate base then cover with the remaining liquid chocolate. Put in the fridge to chill for 10–20 minutes or until hardened.

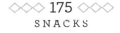

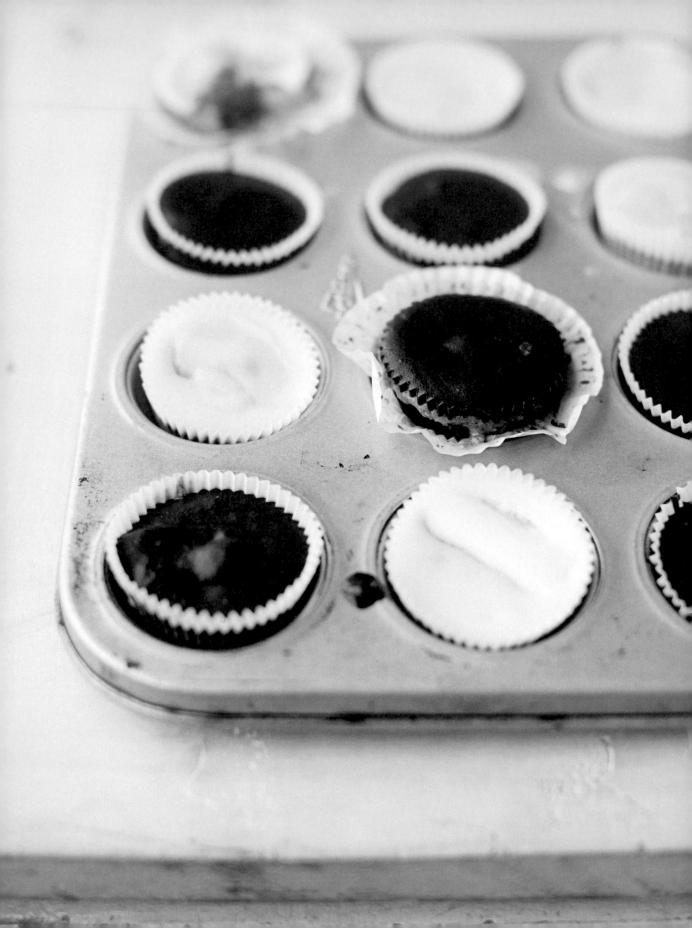

White chocolate nut butter cups

170g (¾ cup) coconut butter
    (not coconut oil)
1 tablespoon pure
    maple syrup
60g (¼ cup) almond butter

White chocolate – say whaaat? OK, I admit – this isn't white chocolate, nor does it taste exactly the same, but it does have a very similar melt-in-the-mouth texture. It's also a great way to get some wonderful healthy fats into your day, helping to produce lots of long-lasting energy!

Start by melting your coconut butter and maple syrup in a pan over a medium heat. Add about 1 teaspoon of the liquid mixture into the bottom of 6 cupcake cases – enough to cover the bottom of each paper case. Put in the freezer for 5 minutes or until the chocolate has hardened.

Remove from the freezer and add 1 teaspoon of almond butter to each coconut and maple base, then cover with the remaining liquid coconut mixture. Put in the fridge to chill for 10–20 minutes or until hardened.

SWITCH IT UP

I love almond butter, but cashew butter or peanut butter would be amazing too in this recipe.

GREEDY FOR GOODNESS?

If you're a superfood addict, and want to give these treats a further nutritional punch, try adding ½ teaspoon of maca or lucuma powder to the white chocolate mix.

Opposite: Nut butter cups and
White chocolate nut butter cups.

Peanut butter bites coated in raw chocolate

MAKES 12–18 BALLS

Peanut butter balls
280g (2 cups) unsalted
 peanuts
180g (1 cup) Medjool
 dates, pitted
¼ teaspoon ground cinnamon

Raw chocolate coating
180ml (¾ cup) melted
 coconut oil
110g (1 cup) raw cacao
 (or cocoa) powder
180ml (¾ cup) agave
 or pure maple syrup

SWITCH IT UP

If you're not a peanut butter
fan, you can switch it up
with almond or cashew butter,
substituting the peanuts
in the recipe with the same
quantity of almonds or
raw cashews.

It's no secret that I'm a total, self-confessed nut butter addict! So, naturally, this recipe is one I completely and utterly adore. It's also super-simple and really fun to make. The raw chocolate coating is incredibly delicious and impossible to resist when you're making it – I always end up with chocolate all over my face!

Preheat the oven to 180°C/160°C fan/gas 4. Scatter the peanuts in a roasting tin and place in the oven to roast for 5–10 minutes until golden brown – shaking once or twice during cooking to ensure they don't burn.

Place the roasted peanuts in a food processor and pulse until coarsely ground – around 30 seconds. Add the dates and cinnamon and process again – for 2–3 minutes. At this point, it's your cue to roll the mixture into balls! Scoop up spoonfuls of the mixture and roll each one between your palms. The mixture makes anything between 12 and 18 balls.

Mix together all the ingredients for the chocolate coating in bowl. Stick a fork into a peanut butter ball and dip it into the chocolate mixture, using a spoon to help coat the ball completely in the chocolate. Repeat with all the balls, placing each one on a plate lined with baking parchment before putting in the freezer to set – this takes about 15 minutes. Once set, transfer to the fridge to store. They will keep like this for up to a week – if you can resist them!

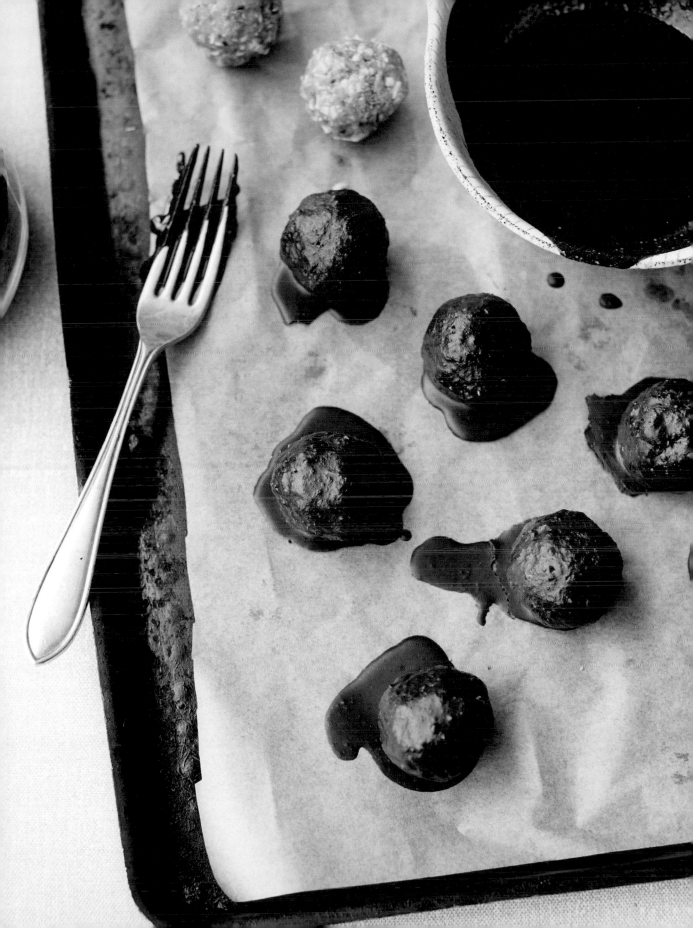

Popcorn – two ways!

**MAKES 1 LARGE BAG
(4 CUPS) POPCORN**

2 tablespoons coconut oil
110g (½ cup) popcorn kernels

Salted chocolate sauce
4 tablespoons coconut
   oil, melted
2 tablespoons pure maple
   syrup
3 tablespoons raw cacao
   (or cocoa) powder
Pinch of salt

Salted caramel sauce
4 tablespoons coconut
   oil, melted
2 tablespoons pure
   maple syrup
2 tablespoons cashew butter
Pinch of salt

I love popcorn – it truly is one of the ultimate movie-night treats. These recipes for two types of sweet-and-salty popcorn are the perfect healthier way to enjoy it.

◇◇◇◇◇◇◇◇◇◇◇◇◇◇◇◇◇◇◇◇◇◇◇◇◇◇◇◇◇◇◇◇◇◇◇◇

Start by putting the coconut oil into a large pan and melting it over a medium heat. Remove from the heat and add your popcorn kernels, then put a lid on the pan and wait 30 seconds before returning to the heat – this allows all the kernels to heat up evenly.

Put the pan back on the heat, with the lid on, and keep on the heat until all the popcorn has finished popping. When all is silent, remove the lid and pour the popcorn into an airtight plastic container.

Now make your sauce of choice. Mix all the ingredients together until smooth, the pour over the popcorn and toss well. Put into the fridge to allow to set for about 15 minutes, or until the sauce has hardened. Stored in an airtight container in the fridge, it will keep for up to 3 days. Uncoated, the popcorn can be kept out of the fridge in an airtight container or resealable plastic bag.

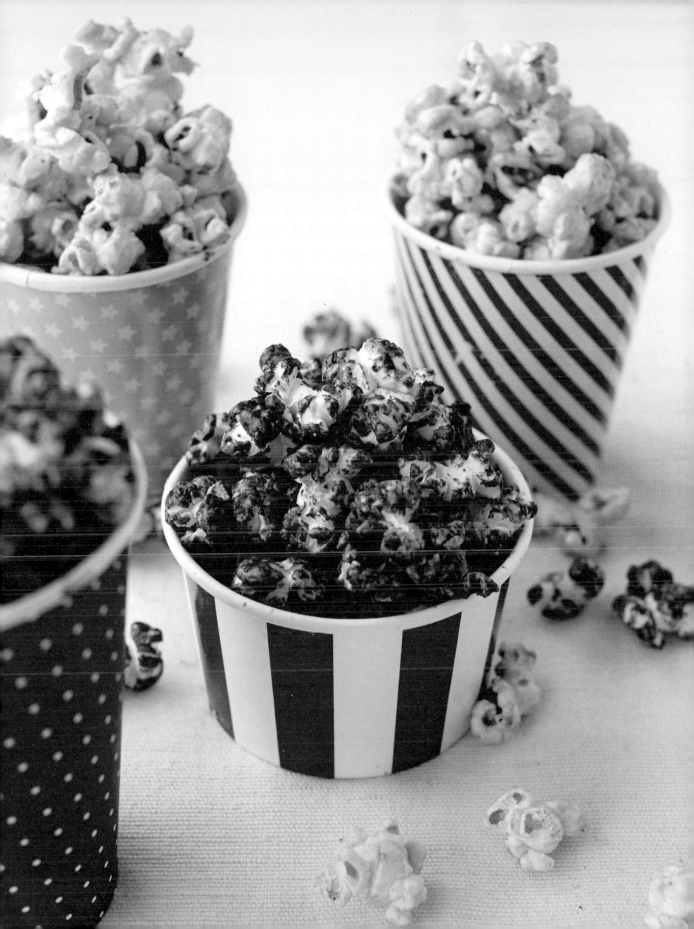

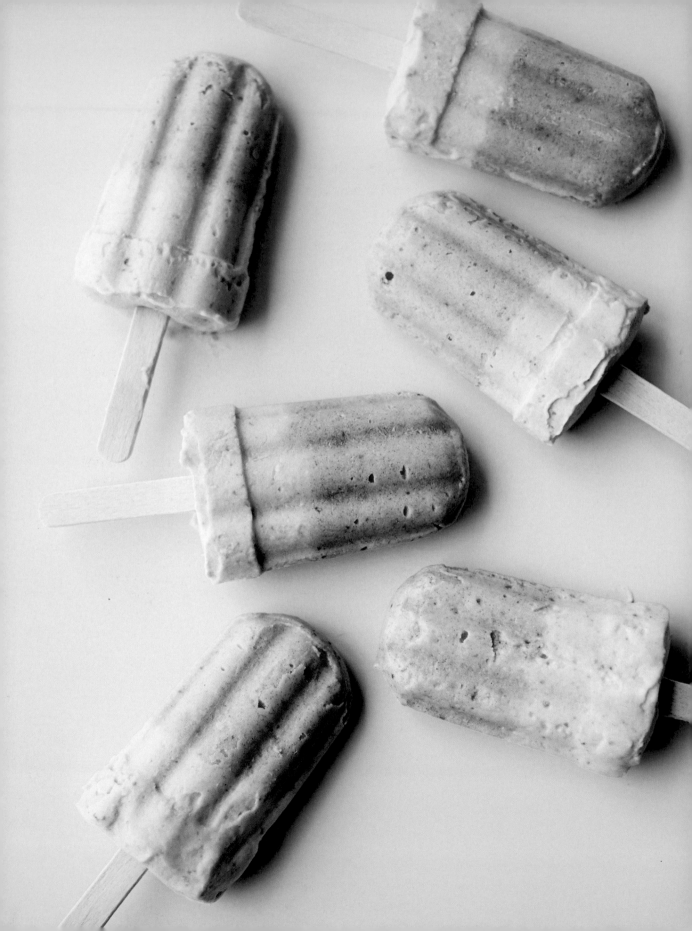

Strawberry and coconut ice-lollies

MAKES 8 ICE-LOLLIES

300ml (1¼ cups) tinned
   full-fat coconut milk
1 banana, peeled
4 Medjool dates, pitted
   and chopped
100g (1 cup) strawberries,
   hulled

I know ice-lollies are a very summery treat, but I love these babies all year round. They're a real saviour when it comes to satisfying those sweet cravings, as I can make lots and keep them in the freezer for ever! I love using other fruit in them, but this particular combination is my favourite.

Place the creamy part of the coconut milk (leaving any watery liquid in the tin) in a blender with the banana and dates and blend until smooth. Pour half the mixture into a jug, add the strawberries to the mixture left in the blender and blend again until smooth.

Pour the strawberry mixture into the ice-lolly moulds and then the remaining coconut mixture on top. Put in the freezer for a couple hours to set.

SWITCH IT UP

Strawberries are my favourite in these ice-lollies, but any sharp-tasting fruit works well: pomegranate seeds, blackberries, blueberries, raspberries – the options are endless.

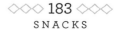

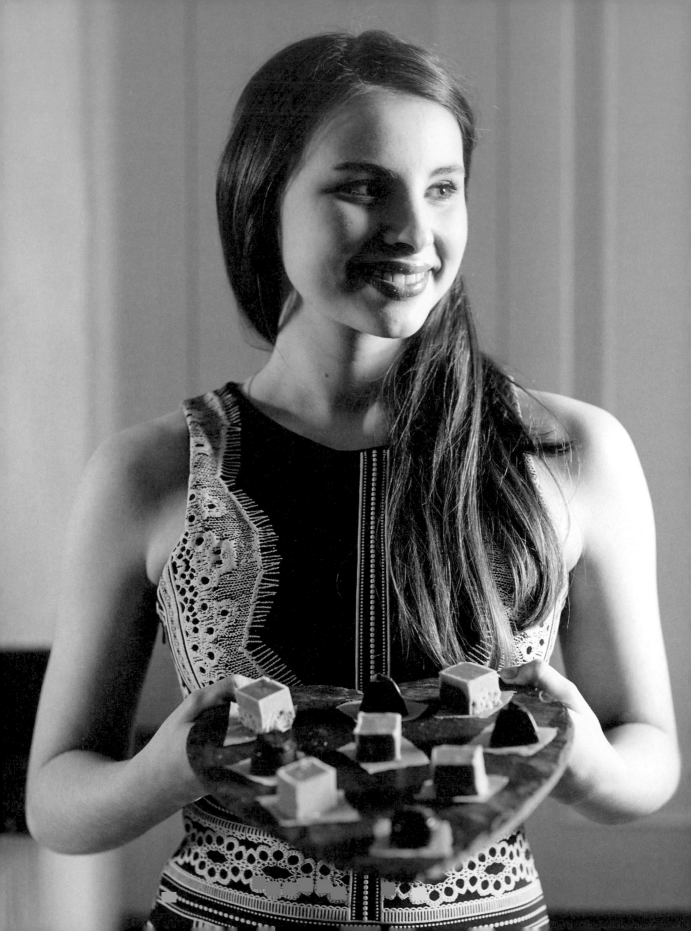

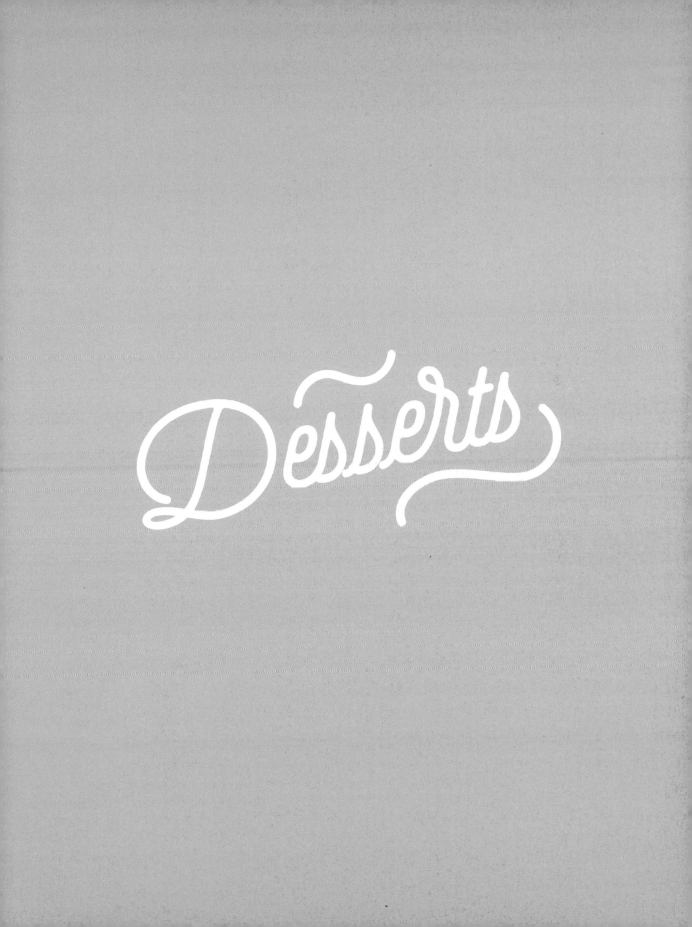

Anyone who knows me knows I've always had a seriously sweet tooth, which was what made the transition to eating such a natural, plant-based diet so daunting!

How could I satisfy my sweet cravings without eating something I would inevitably regret? I was desperate to create recipes that were still really good for you but tasted just as naughty as their unhealthy counterparts. Needless to say, there wasn't a light bulb moment where it all just clicked, and the way to make super-delicious and healthy desserts instantly hit me. Oh no – it took time, practice, lots of washing-up, wasted food and a very messy kitchen! Experimenting with new ingredients and different ways of making dishes really intrigued me, however. It was like learning a whole new vocabulary in the kitchen, and over time it completely changed the way I viewed every meal, my beloved sweet treats included.

This section is packed full of the most deliciously indulgent desserts that you'd never believe were healthy for you – from Sticky toffee pudding and gooey chocolate brownies to Red velvet cupcakes and Raw mango cheesecake (see pages 191, 192, 199 and 200). There's a really balanced range on offer, with lots of fresh fruit, as well as richer chocolate flavours. In case you hadn't noticed, I'm a complete chocoholic!

The ingredients I use for all the recipes are very simple and basic, and because I don't use eggs, sugar or dairy ingredients, they do tend to repeat themselves, which is great, as you can stock up on them, knowing that you'll use them again and again.

I promise that, despite some of the more wacky additions to the recipes (beetroot in the red velvet cupcakes, for example), they all taste identical to their unhealthier counterparts, but with the benefit of your body loving the recipe too! It's really all about making a few simple swaps – replacing the sugar for a natural sweetener, using gluten-free flour, swapping eggs for a little mashed banana, flax or chia seeds and using dairy-free milk and spreads. These simple substitutions will completely change the way your body responds to the meal. No more post-munch slump; instead you'll feel brighter, energised and focused – with a delicious sweet treat into the bargain!

Apple and blueberry crumble with coconut cream

SERVES 6

8 cooking apples
250g (2 cups) blueberries
1 teaspoon ground cinnamon
60ml (¼ cup) water

Topping
200g (2 cups) (gluten-free) rolled oats
120g (1 cup) brown rice flour
2 generous tablespoons coconut oil
80ml (⅓ cup) pure maple syrup
½ tablespoon ground cinnamon

Coconut cream
2 x 400ml tins of full-fat coconut milk
3–4 tablespoons pure maple syrup

I absolutely adore this recipe. There is something so comforting about a bowl of stewed apples and blueberries with hints of cinnamon topped with a wonderful crunchy oat layer. Paired with this incredible coconut cream, it tastes just amazing!

◇◇◇◇◇◇◇◇◇◇◇◇◇◇◇◇◇◇◇◇◇◇◇◇◇◇◇◇◇◇◇◇◇◇◇◇◇

A couple of hours before you start cooking, empty the tins of coconut milk for the coconut cream into an airtight plastic container and place in the freezer. When you're ready to start, remove the container and scoop out the solidified/frozen cream (which will have separated from any watery liquid) into a bowl, allowing it to defrost.

Preheat the oven to 190°C/170°C fan/gas mark 5 and make the topping. Combine the oats and brown rice flour in a mixing bowl. Add the coconut oil, maple syrup and cinnamon to a saucepan and heat until the coconut oil has melted. Pour this into the oat and flour mixture and mix until everything is nicely coated in the syrup, then set aside.

Next peel the apples, removing the core as you go. Slice each into around 10 small chunks – it doesn't matter what shape – and place in a saucepan with the blueberries, cinnamon and water. Simmer over a medium-low heat for 10–15 minutes until the fruit is soft.

Recipe continues overleaf

Recipe continued

While the fruit is cooking, add the defrosted coconut cream to your blender with the maple syrup and blend until smooth. Transfer to a bowl and place in the fridge.

Once the fruit is cooked, pour into the bottom of a baking dish and spread out evenly. Pour the topping over the fruit, making sure to flatten it out in a even layer that covers the fruit entirely. Place in the oven and bake for around 20 minutes, checking after 10 minutes to make sure the topping is golden brown and not burning! (If it's getting too brown, reduce the heat slightly, cover the dish with foil and place on a lower shelf.)

Remove from the oven and serve hot, with a dollop of your amazing coconut cream.

SWITCH IT UP

Blueberries are fantastic in this recipe, but I also like swapping them for blackberries – especially in the early autumn when they're in season and you can either forage for them or buy them really cheaply.

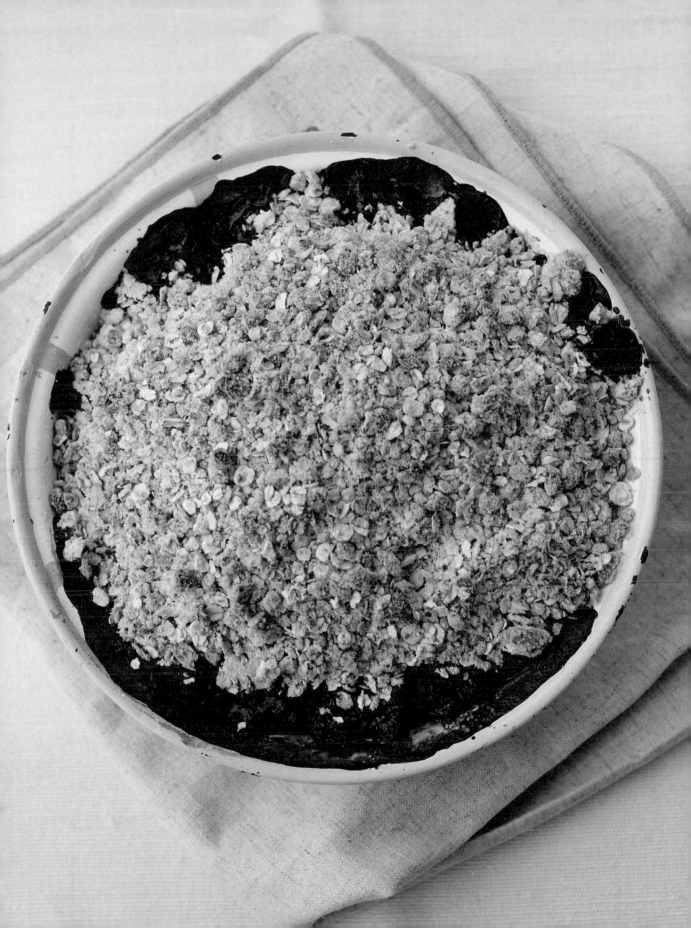

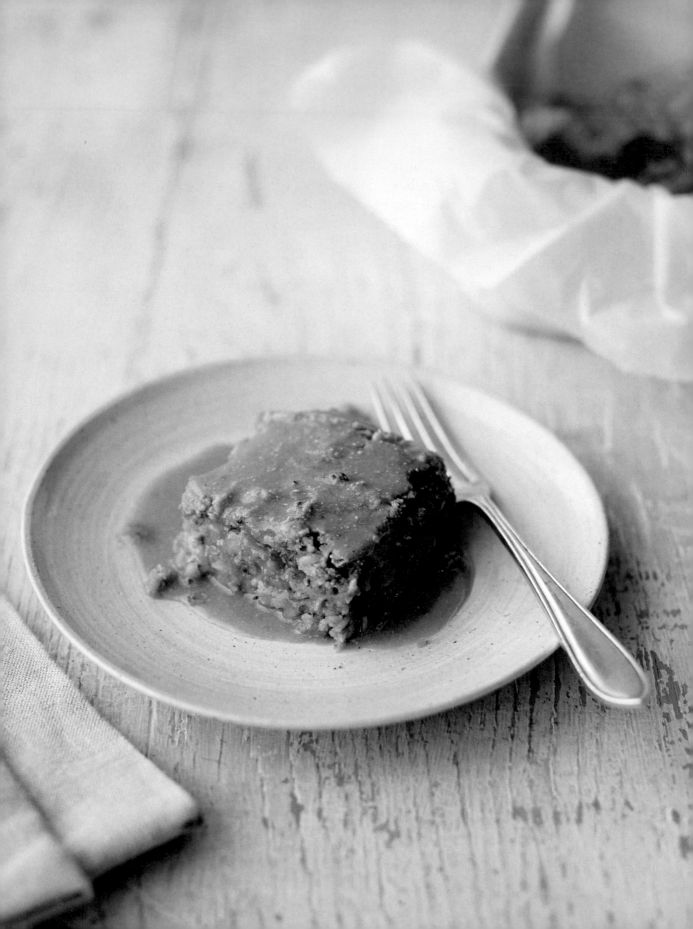

Sticky toffee pudding

SERVES 4

Coconut oil, for greasing
90g (½ cup) Medjool dates,
    pitted and chopped
120ml (½ cup) water
120ml (½ cup) rice milk
150g (1½ cups) (gluten-free)
    rolled oats
3 tablespoons cashew butter
4 tablespoons raw honey
    or agave syrup
2 tablespoons water

I have such fond memories of coming home after school to the smell of sticky toffee pudding wafting from the oven. It was my mum's speciality – much loved by my brother and me. Creating a healthy version the family would approve of was no easy task, but after many failed attempts I finally succeeded! I found a way to recreate all the richness of the classic pudding with really simple, easy and affordable ingredients. It takes no more than 15 minutes to prepare, and will be enjoyed by the whole family.

Preheat the oven to 190°C/170°C fan/gas 5 and grease a 15cm-square baking dish or tin with coconut oil. Add the dates to a saucepan with the water and rice milk. Bring to the boil, then reduce the heat and simmer until the dates start to form a paste with the liquid. Tip in the oats and cook for a further minute.

Stir well, then transfer to the prepared dish or tin, spreading the mixture in an even layer. Place in the oven to bake for 25 minutes.

Meanwhile, stir together the cashew butter and honey or agave syrup with the water. Remove the dish from the oven and pour the cashew and honey/syrup mixture on top of the oats, then put back in the oven to cook for a further 3–5 minutes to heat through until the sauce is piping hot.

Brownies with a salted caramel sauce

80ml (⅓ cup) melted
coconut oil (3 generous
tablespoons before
melting), plus extra
for greasing
40g (¼ cup) chia seeds
180ml (¾ cup) water
270g (1½ cups) Medjool
dates, pitted and chopped
250g (1 cup) nut butter
(I love pecan but you can
use almond, cashew or
peanut – to make your
own, see page 58)
125ml (½ cup) dairy-free
milk of your choice
(to make your own,
see pages 74–75)
120ml (½ cup) pure
maple syrup
120g (1 cup) brown rice flour
55–80g (½–¾ cup) raw cacao
(or cocoa) powder
1 teaspoon baking powder
Pinch of salt

Salted caramel sauce
180g (1 cup) Medjool dates,
pitted and chopped
1–2 tablespoons cashew
or almond butter
60ml (¼ cup) dairy-free milk
of your choice (to make
your own, see pages 74–75)

This recipe is honestly one of the most delicious in the book! It's no trouble at all to prepare, and tastes like a piece of heaven. I'm constantly finding excuses to make these brownies. As my dad would say, 'It's always somebody's birthday somewhere in the world.' Too true! Time to get baking ...

◇◇◇◇◇◇◇◇◇◇◇◇◇◇◇◇◇◇◇◇◇◇◇◇◇◇◇◇◇◇◇◇◇◇

Preheat the oven to 180°C/160°C fan/gas 4, then grease a 20cm-square baking tin with coconut oil and line with baking parchment. In a bowl, combine the chia seeds and the water and leave for 15 minutes.

Put the melted coconut oil in a blender with the dates, nut butter, milk and maple syrup and blend until smooth. Don't worry if its not 100 per cent smooth – a few little pieces of date just add to the texture!

Pour the mixture into a bowl and sift over the remaining ingredients, folding in to combine. Add the soaked chia seeds and mix in well. Tip into the prepared baking tin and place in the oven to bake for around 35 minutes, or until you can insert a skewer or knife into the sponge and it comes out clean.

Meanwhile, make the salted caramel sauce by adding all the ingredients to your blender and blending until smooth. (If the dates are quite hard, it's a good idea to soak them in boiling water for 60 seconds prior to blending, as you don't want any lumps.)

Take the brownies out of the oven and leave to cool. Cut into squares and serve with the caramel sauce – either as it is or heated up – drizzled over.

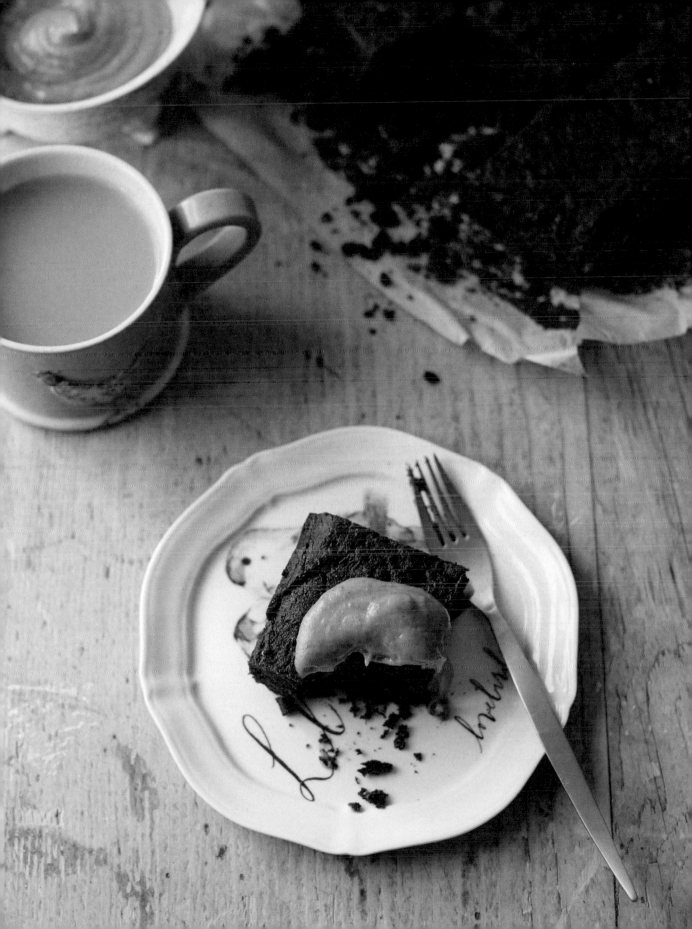

Banoffee pie

5 bananas, peeled, plus
   2 bananas to decorate
120g (½ cup) almond butter
5 Medjool dates, pitted
   and chopped
180ml (¾ cup) dairy-free
   milk (almond, oat or rice)
Cacao nibs, finely grated,
   for sprinkling

Base
Coconut oil, for greasing
240g (2 cups) cashews
180g (1 cup) Medjool dates,
   pitted and chopped
1 tablespoon water
3 tablespoons raw cacao (or
   cocoa) powder (optional)

Coconut cream
2 x 400ml tins of full-fat
   coconut milk
60ml (¼ cup) pure
   maple syrup

Everyone who's tried this absolutely adores it, and can't believe that it's actually healthy for you. This dessert, unlike its sugar-laden counterparts, will leave you feeling light and energised.

◇◇◇◇◇◇◇◇◇◇◇◇◇◇◇◇◇◇◇◇◇◇◇◇◇◇◇◇◇◇◇◇◇◇

A couple of hours before you start, empty the tins of coconut milk for the coconut cream into an airtight plastic container and place in the freezer. When you're ready to start, remove the container and scoop out the solidified cream (which will have separated from any watery liquid) into a bowl. Leave to defrost.

Start by making the base. Grease a 20cm-diameter flan dish or loose-bottomed tart tin with coconut oil, then grind the cashews in a food processor until they form a fine flour. Pour into a bowl and add the dates, water and cacao (or cocoa) powder (if using). Stir into a paste, then use your hands to combine into a dough. Mould into the bottom of the prepared tart tin, pushing partway up the sides of the tin. Place in the fridge to set.

Add the bananas to your blender with the almond butter, dates and milk and blend until smooth. Pour onto the set base and place in the freezer for at least 2 hours to harden. Meanwhile, add the defrosted coconut cream to a blender with the maple syrup and blend until smooth. Pour into a bowl and leave to set.

When you're almost ready to eat, remove the pie from the freezer and transfer from the tin to a serving plate. Allow it to thaw before adding slices of banana on top, followed by dollops of the cream and a sprinkling of finely grated cacao nibs.

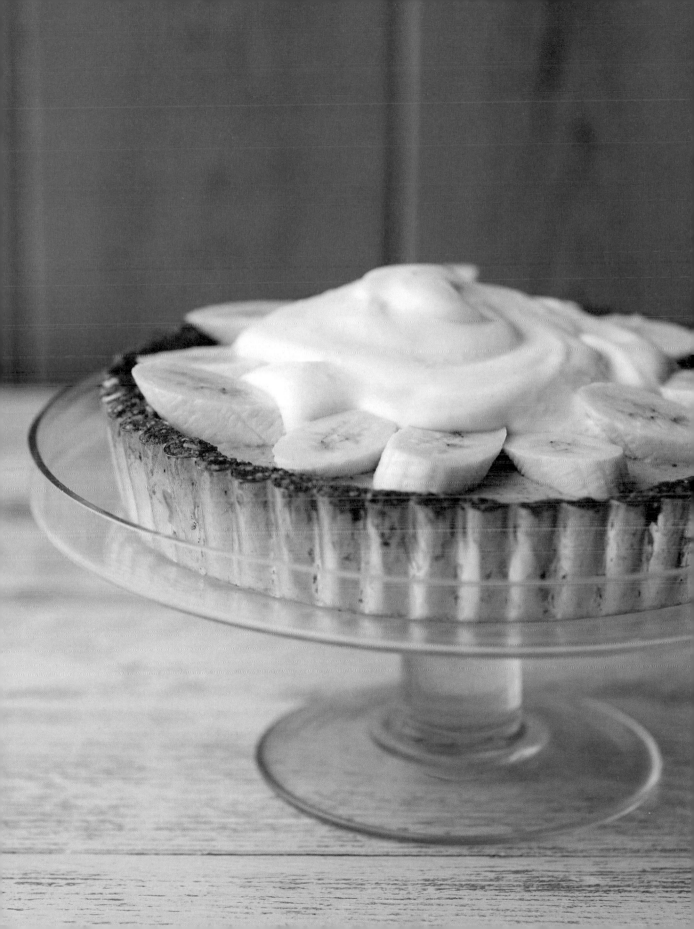

Light and fluffy chocolate cake with chocolate frosting

SERVES 6–8

120ml (½ cup) olive oil or melted coconut oil, plus extra for greasing
300g (3 cups) ground almonds
55g (½ cup) raw cacao (or cocoa) powder
2 teaspoons baking powder
1 banana, peeled and mashed
120ml (½ cup) oat or almond milk
5 tablespoons raw honey, agave or pure maple syrup

Chocolate frosting
180g (1 cup) Medjool dates, pitted and chopped
30g (¼ cup) raw cacao (or cocoa) powder
2 generous tablespoons coconut oil, melted
120ml (½ cup) water

To decorate (optional)
Dessicated coconut
Dried goji berries
Slices of fresh strawberry
Cacao nibs

TIP

For the frosting, make sure you use Medjool as opposed to regular dates. These don't blend as well, and so the icing will be much lumpier. If you are using regular dates, it's best to soak them in boiling water for 5 minutes, or until really soft.

I've experimented with a fair few vegan chocolate cakes in my time, and none of them really hit the spot – they can be too fudgy and very dense. This one is an exception, proving that a chocolate cake made with healthy ingredients can also be light, fluffy and just the right moist texture.

Preheat the oven to 180°C/160°C fan/gas 4, then grease an 18cm-diameter loose-bottomed cake tin with olive/coconut oil and line the base with baking parchment. In a mixing bowl, combine the ground almonds, cacao (or cocoa) powder and baking powder. Add the mashed banana, oil, milk and honey or agave/ maple syrup and mix well to form a smooth batter.

Spoon the mixture into your prepared cake tin, smoothing over the top, and place in the oven to bake for about 40 minutes, checking after half an hour, until well risen and cooked through – a skewer or point of a knife inserted into the cake should come out clean.

While the cake is cooking, make the frosting. Add all ingredients to your blender and blend until smooth! Place in a bowl and store in the fridge until needed.

Remove the cake from the oven and leave to cool in the tin for 5 minutes, then transfer to a wire rack and allow to cool completely. Once cooled, spread the frosting over the top of the cake and decorate, if you like, with your choice of topping. I love using edible white flowers if I can find them!

SWITCH IT UP

For anyone who doesn't have a blender to make the frosting, try this simple recipe. Place 250g (1 cup) nut butter (cashew, almond or peanut) in a bowl with 4 tablespoons maple syrup, 2 tablespoons raw cacao (or cocoa) powder and 2 tablespoons dairy-free milk. Mix everything together and put in the fridge to thicken.

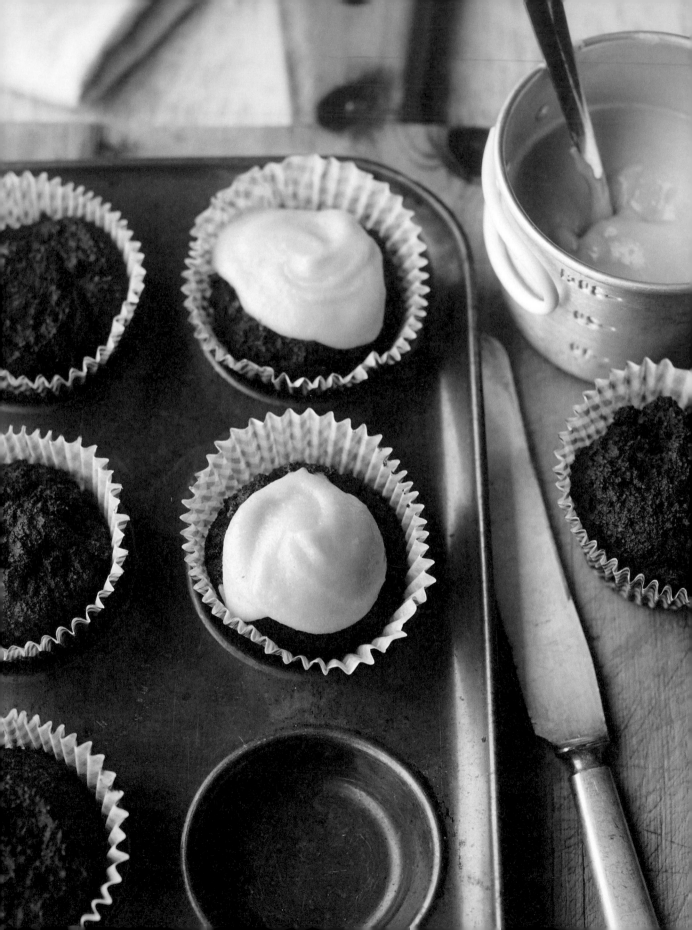

Red velvet cupcakes with a cashew 'buttercream' icing

MAKES 12 CUPCAKES

60ml (¼ cup) olive oil
    or melted coconut oil
150g (1½ cups) ground
    almonds
30g (¼ cup) raw cacao
    (or cocoa) powder
1 teaspoon baking powder
½ banana, peeled and mashed
60ml (¼ cup) beetroot juice
2 tablespoons raw honey,
    agave or pure maple syrup

'Buttercream' icing
120g (1 cup) cashews,
    soaked in water for at
    least 2 hours or overnight
1 tablespoon lemon juice
60ml (¼ cup) pure
    maple syrup
2 tablespoons coconut
    oil, melted

Growing up in the USA, I have some foodie memories that remain really vivid, such as my weekly red velvet cupcake stop before ballet class. I love red velvet cupcakes, and it became a routine to buy one. As with most of my recipes, I aim to create healthier versions of the naughty foods I adored as a child. This recipe tastes just as delicious as the red velvet cupcakes I used to enjoy, but is packed with good ingredients that, instead of making you feel bloated and lethargic, give you more energy and focus to help see you through the day.

Preheat the oven to 180°C/160° fan/gas 4, then line a 12-hole bun tin with paper cases or grease 12 individual cupcake tins with coconut oil. In a mixing bowl, combine the ground almonds, cacao (or cocoa) powder and baking powder. Add the banana, oil, beetroot juice and honey, agave or maple syrup and mix well to form a smooth batter.

Spoon into the paper cases or individual tins and bake in the oven for 25 minutes until well risen and cooked through. Remove from the oven, allow to cool in the tin (or tins) for 5 minutes, then transfer to a wire rack to cool down fully.

For the 'buttercream', drain the soaked cashews and add all the ingredients to a high-powered blender or food processor, blending until smooth. Once the cupcakes have cooled, generously top each of them with your buttercream in a nice thick layer.

Raw mango cheesecake with a chocolate brownie base

SERVES 8

Chocolate base
230g (2 cups) pecans
180g (1 cup) Medjool
    dates, pitted
3 tablespoons raw cacao
    (or cocoa) powder
⅛ teaspoon salt (preferably
    pink Himalayan)

Mango topping
4 generous tablespoons
    coconut oil, melted,
    plus extra for greasing
240g (2 cups) cashews,
    soaked in water for at
    least 2 hours or overnight,
    then drained
2 mangos, peeled and stoned
60ml (¼ cup) pure
    maple syrup

I'm a big fan of raw cakes, and this one beats them all. The combination of cashews and mango makes the most unbelievably creamy mix. The flavour coming through from the base is incredibly chocolatey, which enhances the lighter, fruitier taste of the topping. I'm a bit of an addict as far as this cheesecake is concerned, and tend to sneak far too much from the blender before the dish is even finished!

Start by greasing a 20cm-diameter spring-form cake tin with coconut oil. To make the chocolate base, first add the pecans to a food processor and pulse into a fine crumb. Add the dates, cacao (or cocoa) powder and salt and process again until the mixture has formed a raw 'dough'. Press into the bottom of the prepared cake tin to form an even layer.

Add all the ingredients for the topping to the food processor or a high-powered blender and blend until smooth. Pour on top of the base and spread out evenly. Place the finished cheesecake in the freezer to set for 1–2 hours. Once set, remove from the freezer, carefully transfer from the tin to a plate and allow to thaw. Simply slice and serve!

SWITCH IT UP

You don't have to use mango to make a delicious dairy-free cheesecake – try this recipe using any fruit you prefer or have to hand. Blueberries, raspberries or strawberries work a treat, for instance.

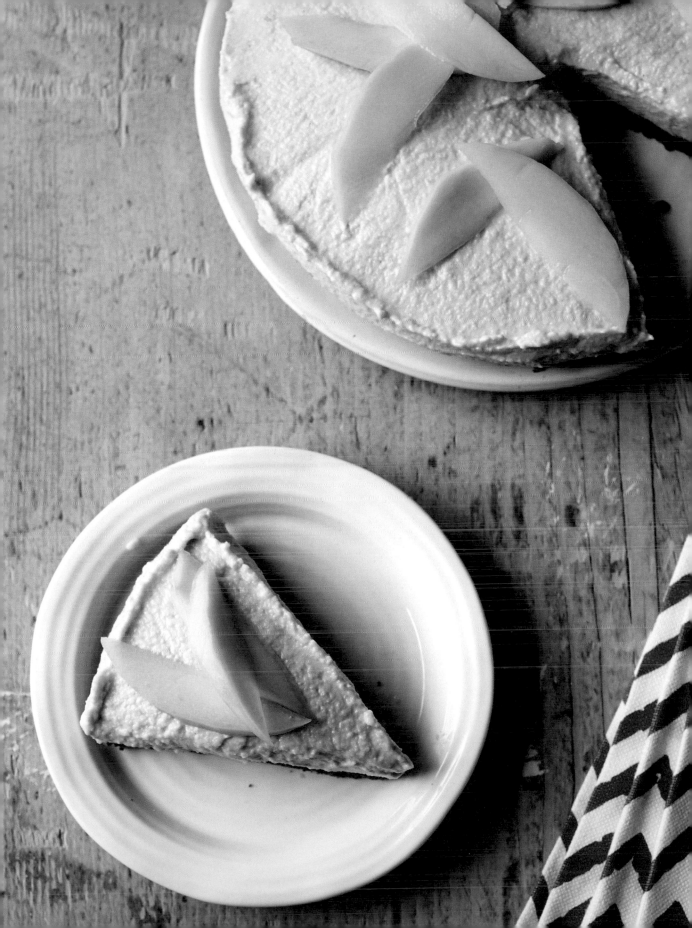

Poached pears with a chocolate sauce and vanilla ice cream

SERVES 2

Poached pears
Zest of 1 lemon
1 cinnamon stick
1 vanilla bean (split
    lengthways – optional)
¼ teaspoon ground allspice
240ml (1 cup) apple
    cider vinegar
2 pears, peeled and kept
    whole, retaining the stalks

Vanilla ice cream
120g (1 cup) cashews, soaked
    in water for at least 2 hours
    or overnight, then drained
2 tablespoons coconut
    oil, melted
1 tablespoon agave syrup
Seeds from ½ vanilla pod
120ml (½ cup) water

Chocolate sauce
4 tablespoons coconut
    oil, melted
2 tablespoons pure
    maple syrup
3 tablespoons raw cacao
    (or cocoa) powder

SWITCH IT UP
Instead of pears, you could
poach apples and serve with a
caramel sauce (see page 192),
in addition to the ice cream.

My favourite desserts tend to be the heavy-duty ones like chocolate brownies, cheesecakes and mousses – puddings that, while made with healthy ingredients, taste über-rich and indulgent. This dish is much lighter, fresher and fruitier and, although unlike my normal 'go to' for puds, has become a real favourite.

◇◇◇◇◇◇◇◇◇◇◇◇◇◇◇◇◇◇◇◇◇◇◇◇◇◇◇◇◇◇◇

First make the ice cream. Add all the ingredients to a high-powered blender or food processor and blend! Pour into a freezer-proof plastic container and place in the freezer for 5–6 hours to set.

To poach the pears, first place the lemon zest in a saucepan with the cinnamon stick, vanilla pod, allspice, water and vinegar. Bring to a simmer and add the pears. Leave to poach for 20 minutes, or until the pears have softened slightly, turning the pears occasionally.

When the pears are cooked, use a slotted spoon to transfer them to a bowl, then place to one side. Increase the temperature of the poaching liquid and bring to the boil, continuing to boil until it has reduced to a syrup – roughly 10 minutes. Pour the syrup over the pears.

Combine all the ingredients for the chocolate sauce in a small bowl, leaving it as it is or heating through, if you prefer. Place the poached pears in individual bowls, pour over the sauce and serve with a scoop of vanilla ice cream. (The ice cream makes much more than you'll need – you can store the rest in the freezer to enjoy another time!)

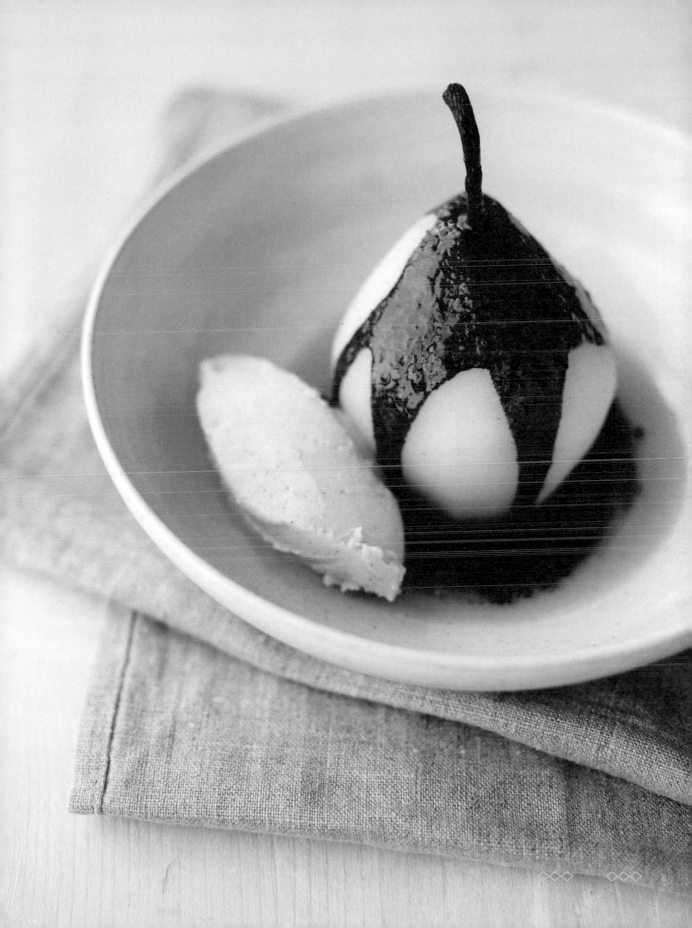

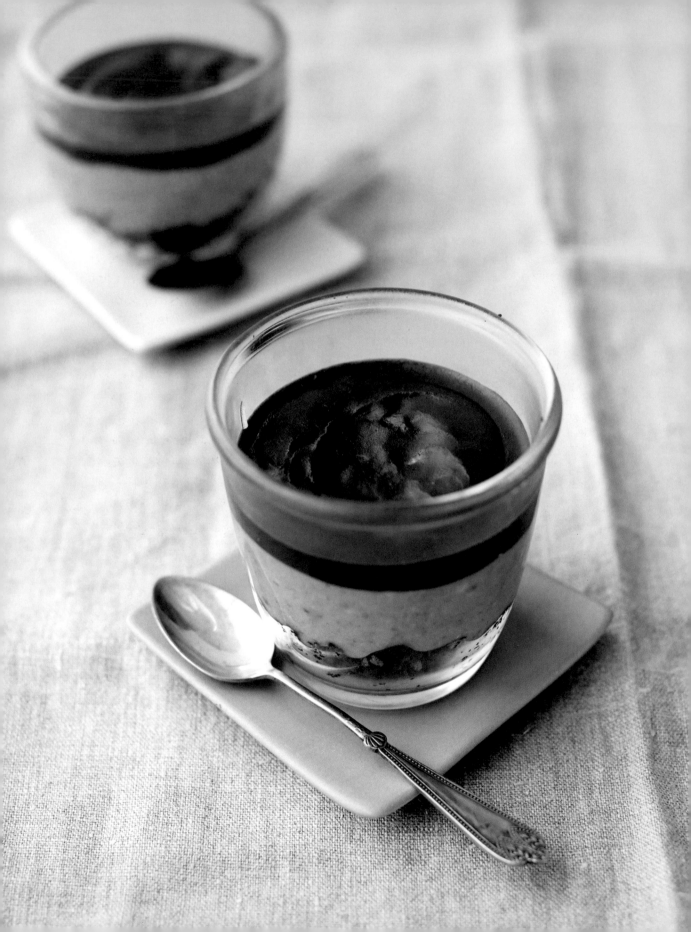

Caramel mousse with a raw chocolate ganache

MAKES 2 MOUSSES

Base
115g (1 cup) pecans
3 tablespoons raw cacao
   (or cocoa) powder
90g (⅓ cup) Medjool
   dates, pitted
Pinch of salt

Caramel layer
125g (½ cup) cashew butter
45g (¼ cup) Medjool dates,
   pitted and chopped
2 tablespoons coconut
   oil, melted
1 tablespoon raw honey,
   agave or pure maple syrup
½ teaspoon ground cinnamon
60–120ml (¼–½ cup) water
   (start with less and add
   more if needed)

Raw chocolate ganache
2 generous tablespoons
   coconut oil, melted
30g (¼ cup) raw cacao
   (or cocoa) powder
80ml (¼ cup) agave or
   maple syrup

Despite being made from completely natural ingredients, this is one of the most indulgent desserts I have ever tasted. The base consists of a fudge brownie, with a hint of sweet pecan and a subtle caramel overtone from the Medjool dates. The middle is like a caramel mousse with hints of cinnamon and coconut. To top it all is a layer of raw chocolate ganache – sheer heaven!

Make the base by adding the pecans and cacao (or cocoa) powder to a food processor and process into a fine flour, then add the dates and blend again until it becomes a sticky dough. Divide the dough in two and press into the bottom of a glass or jar.

Make the caramel layer by adding all ingredients to a blender and blending until smooth. Pour on top of the base in each glass or jar.

To make the chocolate chocolate ganache, mix all the ingredients until smooth, then pour the chocolate on top of the caramel layer and place in the fridge to chill until you are ready to serve.

Banana ice cream – three ways!

Strawberry
50g (½ cup) frozen
    strawberries
2 bananas, peeled, sliced
    and frozen
2 tablespoons dairy-free milk
    of your choice (to make
    your own, see pages 74–75)

Chocolate
3 bananas, peeled, sliced
    and frozen
1 tablespoon raw cacao
    (or cocoa) powder
1 tablespoon agave or
    pure maple syrup
Cacao nibs, for sprinkling
    on top

Honeycomb
3 bananas, peeled, sliced
    and frozen
1 tablespoon raw honey,
    agave or pure maple syrup
1 tablespoon almond butter
Chopped-up pecans, for
    sprinkling on top

Banana ice cream is a super-simple way to get your sweet fix. All you have to do is blend frozen bananas with your flavour of choice and, voilà, you've got an incredibly decadent and flavour-packed ice cream that's actually really good for you.

For each of the three options, add everything (minus the toppings) to a high-powered blender or a food processor and blend until smooth. These are best served straight away, sprinkled with the topping, though they can be stored in a container in the freezer for up to 2 weeks.

SWITCH IT UP

Experiment with different flavours, using the same base of frozen banana. Frozen mango, raspberries or blueberries would all work well. I'm also a fan of adding pure vanilla extract and a little cinnamon.

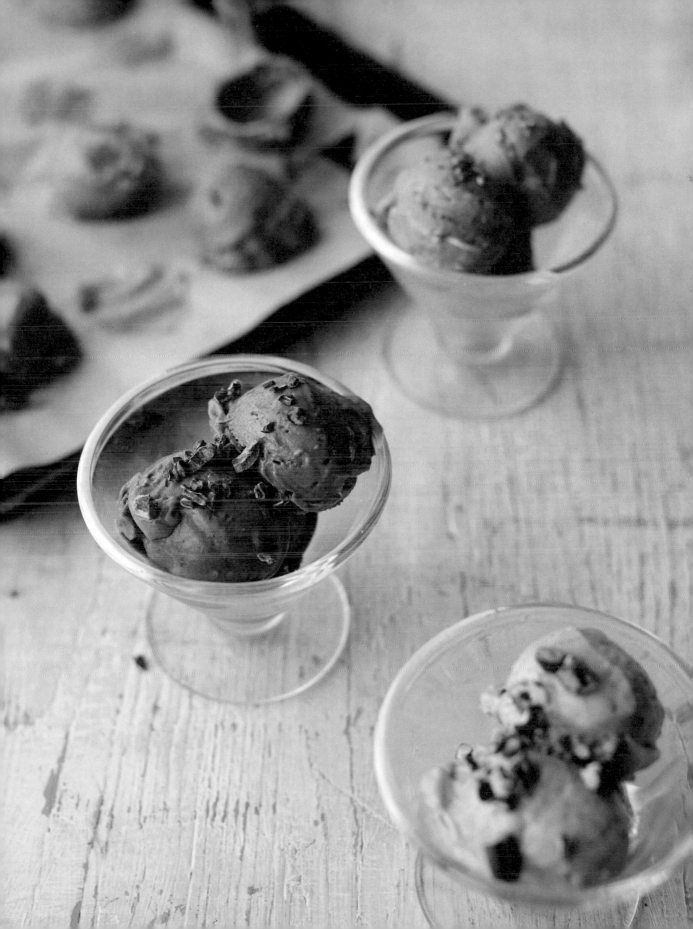

Peanut butter and cinnamon fudge

MAKES 8–12 PIECES

3 generous tablespoons
    coconut oil
225g (1 cup) peanut butter
4 tablespoons agave or
    pure maple syrup
Pinch of ground cinnamon

TIPS

Make sure the peanut butter
has no added sugar, and is
made of only two or three
ingredients: peanuts, a pinch
of salt and maybe a little oil.

This fudge needs to be kept
in the fridge or it will melt
very quickly! My alternative
name for it is 'freezer fudge'
as that's where I like to
keep it.

This peanut butter fudge is beyond delicious, and
another recipe that's quick as anything to make. It
melts in your mouth and tastes incredibly naughty!
(See photo on page 184).

Melt your coconut oil and add to a mixing bowl with
all the other ingredients. Stir into a very smooth paste,
then pour into a 12cm x 18cm plastic container. Place
in the freezer for 30 minutes to set, then slice into
little squares and enjoy!

Raw chocolates

**MAKES AROUND
12 CHOCOLATES**

110g (1 cup) raw cacao
(or cocoa) powder
4 tablespoons agave or
pure maple syrup
4 generous tablespoons
coconut oil, melted

TIP

These chocolates need
to be kept in the fridge,
so don't leave them out
too long or they'll melt!

This recipe for healthy chocolate uses only three,
easy-to-find, natural ingredients: coconut oil, raw
cacao (or cocoa) powder and your choice of either
pure maple or agave syrup. You will also need a
chocolate mould, but if you don't want to buy one
or simply can't wait because you want to make them
right now, then you can set the chocolate in ice-cube
moulds, or pop a tablespoonful into a few muffin
cases before putting them on a plate or tray in the
fridge. This recipe takes around 5 minutes to make
and it's the perfect answer to those sweet cravings!
(See photo on page 184).

Start by placing the cacao (or cocoa) powder in a bowl
with the agave or maple syrup. Add the coconut oil to
the bowl, stirring until the chocolate is smooth. Pour
the mixture into your chocolate moulds and place in
the fridge to set for about 15 minutes before removing
from the moulds.

3-DAY MEAL PLANS

The best thing about eating such nutrient-rich food is the way you can gear it to suit you personally, whatever your lifestyle. Different meals work best for different people and meals can be designed to complement whatever you are doing each day. With this in mind, I've put together a collection of sample meal plans, over a 3-day period, to cover a range of lifestyles, from 'Gym Bunnies' to 'Everyday Eats', or to give that extra bit of help if you're feeling at a low ebb or need to lose weight. Additional recipe suggestions are supplied below each plan. These are just to get you going – to give an idea of how to combine my recipes and help kick-start the healthiest, happiest you!

Gym Bunnies

They say abs are made in the kitchen, not the gym, which is partly true, as nutrition plays a big part in the way your body looks. As a gym-goer and ballet dancer, I know the importance of fuelling yourself with the right foods. This meal plan is all about feeding yourself fit, and helping your muscles recover pre- and post-workout.

Breakfast: Quinoa and Chia Bread (page 63) with Nut Butter (page 58)
Lunch: Kale Salad with Maple Roasted Walnuts, Cranberries and Citrus-sesame Dressing (page 92)
Dinner: Quinoa with Orange-Chilli Kale and Roasted Butternut Squash (page 146)
Snack: Raw Chocolate Brownie Bar (page 172)

Breakfast: Chickpea 'Crêpe' with Tomatoes and Mushrooms (page 36)
Lunch: Lemon-Infused Wild Rice with Parsley, Dried Apricots and Pistachios (page 104)
Dinner: Turmeric-roasted Cauliflower, Garlic Rice and Tahini-Cumin Sauce (page 136)
Snack: Trail Mix (page 171)

Breakfast: Chocolate Overnight Oats with Crushed Raspberries and Coconut (page 48)
Lunch: Beetroot and Butternut Soup (page 88)
Dinner: Lentil Cottage Pie with Sweet Potato Mash (page 154)
Dessert: Peanut Butter and Cinnamon Fudge (page 208)

Recipes to Pick and Mix
Breakfast: Berry-Creamy Smoothie Bowl (page 34); Chocolate Porridge (page 44); Almond, Cinnamon and Banana Porridge with a Blueberry Compote (page 41); Overnight Oats of your choice (pages 46–47); On-the-go Breakfast Sandwiches of your choice (page 55); Baked Carrot Cake Oatmeal (page 27)
Lunch: Lemon Quinoa Tabbouleh with Carrot, Red Pepper and Avocado (page 96); Mexican Slaw with Tamari Vinaigrette and Roasted Cashews (page 99); Brown Rice Pasta Salad with Avocado, Rocket and Pesto Vinaigrette (page 106); Pesto-Courgette Ribbons, Roasted Squash and Tamari Pumpkin Seeds (page 97); Sweet Potato and Leek Soup with Chilli-Roasted Seeds (page 89)

Dinner: Mexican Quinoa, Guacamole and Soured Cream Parfait (page 153); Sweet Potato and Spinach Dhal with Chickpea Naan Bread (page 141); Vegan Enchiladas (page 134); Spicy Squash and Black Bean Burgers (page 144)

Snacks: Energising Berry-Cashew Smoothie (page 78); Peanut Butter Bites Coated in Raw Chocolate (page 178); Raw Gingerbread Bars (page 172); Sticky Almond Butter Flapjacks (page 174)

Speedy Gonzales

When I know I have a busy week ahead, I like to have a quick think through what I'll be eating to ensure I'm stocked up on enough good wholesome ingredients. This meal plan is for the busy bee, and is all about meals that are both nourishing and very quick and easy to make.

Breakfast: Berry-Creamy Smoothie Bowl (page 34)
Lunch: A selection of 'Food on the Go' (pages 109–111)
Dinner: Courgette Noodles with a Sun-Dried Tomato Sauce and Sautéed Mushrooms (page 125)
Snack: Trail Mix (page 171)

Breakfast: Banoffee Overnight Oats (page 45)
Lunch: A selection of 'Food on the Go' (pages 109–111)
Dinner: Hummus and Black Bean Quesadillas (page 130)
Dessert: Banana Ice Cream (page 206)

Breakfast: Avocado, Tomato, Onion and Lemon with Gluten-Free Bread (page 55)
Lunch: A selection of 'Food on the Go' (pages 109–111)
Dinner: Spiced Carrot, Coriander and Chickpea Fritters (page 129)
Sweet Treat: Raw Chocolates (page 209)

Extra Recipes to Pick and Mix
Breakfast: Smoothie Bowl of your choice (pages 28–31); Overnight Oats of your choice (pages 46–47); Coconut Chia Pudding with Crushed Raspberries (page 52); On-the-go Breakfast Sandwiches (page 55); Flax and Goji Berry Muesli (page 65)
Lunch: A selection of 'Food on the Go' (pages 109–111)
Dinner: Pho Courgette Noodle Soup (page 116); Creamy One-Pot Pasta (page 119); Pad Thai (page 122); Tomato and Chilli Stir-Fry with Lemon-Infused Quinoa (page 126)
Snacks: Raw Gingerbread Bars (page 172)

Detoxer

This meal plan is aimed at anyone who wants to re-energise and cleanse their body, lose weight and kick-start a healthier way of life. The meals are packed full of nutrient-rich smoothies, thick and creamy soups and lots of anti-inflammatory veggies.

Breakfast: Coconut Chia Pudding with Crushed Raspberries (page 52)
Lunch: Avocado Gazpacho (page 91)
Dinner: Pho Courgette Noodle Soup (page 116)
Snack: Kale Crisps (page 168)

Breakfast: Gingerbread Smoothie (page 79)
Lunch: Baby Leaf, Pomegranate, Avocado
and Sweet Potato Salad with an Orange
Dressing (page 103)
Dinner: Sweet Potato and Leek Soup with
Chilli-Roasted Seeds (page 89)
Snack: The Perfect Green Juice (page 80)

Breakfast: Glowing Green Smoothie
(page 32)
Lunch: Spicy Red Pepper Soup (page 87)
Dinner: Pad Thai (page 122)

Extra Recipes to Pick and Mix
Breakfast: Smoothie Bowl of your choice
(pages 28–31); Berry Burst Smoothie
(page 82); Anti-Inflammatory Gingerbread
Smoothie (page 79); Flax and Goji Berry
Muesli (page 65)
Lunch: Kale Salad with Maple Roasted
Walnuts, Cranberries and Citrus-sesame
Dressing (page 92); Pesto-Courgette
Ribbons, Roasted Squash Salad and Tamari
Pumpkin Seeds (page 97); Beetroot, Lentil
and Pine Nut Salad with a Balsamic Lemon
Vinaigrette (page 93); Lemon Quinoa
Tabbouleh with Carrot, Red Pepper and
Avocado (page 96); Spicy Red Pepper Soup
(page 87); Avocado Gazpacho (page 91)
Dinner: Courgette Noodles with a Sun-Dried
Tomato Sauce and Sautéed Mushrooms
(page 125); Sweet Potato and Spinach Dhal
with Chickpea Naan Bread (page 141);
Moroccan Root Tagine and Cauliflower
Couscous (page 139); Tomato and Chilli
Stir-Fry with Lemon-Infused Quinoa
(page 126)
Snacks: Raw Gingerbread Bars (page 172)

Body Booster

This meal plan is all about building your
body up, making it stronger, and helping start
the journey to a much healthier you. When
needing to feed your body, such as after
a bout of illness or if you're an endurance
athlete preparing for a big event, it can be
just as hard, both mentally and physically,
as trying to lose weight. It's all about snacking
regularly, and having really rich, nutrient-
dense meals with lots of healthy fats like
those contained in avocados, coconut, nuts
and seeds. The plan below is a general guide
to the sort of foods that will make you feel
amazing and give your body everything
it needs.

Breakfast: Mango and Cashew Overnight
Oats (page 50) and Matcha Latte (page 76)
Snack: Trail Mix (page 171)
Lunch: Brown Rice Pasta Salad with Avocado,
Rocket and Pesto Vinaigrette (page 106)
Snack: Raw Gingerbread Bars (page 172)
Dinner: Creamy Butternut Squash and
Sage Risotto (page 149)
Snack: Flax and Goji Berry Muesli (page 65)
with dairy-free milk

Breakfast: Banoffee Overnight Oats
(page 45)
Snack: Sticky Almond Butter Flapjacks
(page 174)
Lunch: Lemon-Infused Wild Rice with
Parsley, Dried Apricots and Pistachios
(page 104)
Snack: Trail Mix (page 171)
Dinner: Ratatouille Pasta with Brazil Nut
Parmesan (page 150)
Snack: Flax and Goji Berry Muesli (page 65)
with dairy-free milk

Breakfast: Coconut and Raspberry Porridge
(page 42) with sliced banana
Snack: Raw Chocolate Brownie Bars
(page 172)
Lunch: Kale Salad with Maple Roasted
Walnuts, Cranberries and Citrus-sesame
Dressing (page 92)
Snack: Hummus (page 165) with Gluten-
Free Poppy Seed Crackers (page 169)
Dinner: Chilli Non-Carne with Spicy Baked
Potato Wedges and Guacamole (page 131)

Extra Recipes to Pick and Mix
Breakfast: Banana Pancakes with a Blueberry
Syrup (page 59); Golden Granola and
Coconut Cream Parfait (page 66);
Chocolate Porridge (page 44); Mango and
Cashew Overnight Oats (page 50)
Lunch: Coconut Rice with a Mango and
Avocado Salsa (page 120); Mexican Quinoa,
Guacamole and Soured Cream Parfait
(page 153)
Dinner: Creamy Butternut Squash and Sage
Risotto (page 149); Creamy One-Pot Pasta,
(page 119); Chilli Non-Carne with Spicy
Baked Potato Wedges and Guacamole
(page 131)
Snacks: Root Vegetable Crisps (page 170);
Hummus (page 165) and Gluten-Free
Poppy Seed Crackers (page 169); Peanut
Butter Bites Coated in Raw Chocolate
(page 178)

Everyday Eats

Sometimes there is no occasion to prepare
for, other than just eating well on an everyday
basis. These recipes are quick to make and
delicious – perfect for a one-size portion,
or multiplied to feed the whole family.

Breakfast: Flax and Goji Berry Muesli
(page 65) with dairy-free milk
Lunch: A selection of 'Food on the Go'
(pages 109–111)
Dinner: Sweet Potato and Spinach Dhal
with Chickpea Naan Bread (page 141)

Breakfast: Chocolate Porridge (page 44)
Lunch: Pesto-Courgette Ribbons, Roasted
Squash Salad and Tamari Pumpkin Seeds
(page 97)
Dinner: Creamy One-Pot Pasta (page 119)

Breakfast: Quinoa and Chia Bread (page 63),
toasted, with Raspberry and Chia Jam
(page 57)
Lunch: Mexican Slaw with Tamari
Vinaigrette and Roasted Cashews (page 99)
Dinner: Tomato and Chilli Stir-Fry with
Lemon-Infused Quinoa (page 126)

Extra Recipes to Pick and Mix
Breakfast: Smoothie Bowl of your choice
(pages 28–31); Chickpea 'Crêpe' with
Tomatoes and Mushrooms (page 36);
Porridge of your choice (pages 38–39);
Golden Granola (page 66);
Lunch: A selection of 'Food on the Go'
(pages 109–111); your choice of salads
or soups (pages 87–106)
Dinner: Vegan Enchiladas (page 134);
Turmeric-Roasted Cauliflower, Garlic Rice
and Tahini-Cumin Sauce (page 136); Chilli
Non-Carne with Spicy Baked Potato Wedges
and Guacamole (page 131); Spiced Carrot,
Coriander and Chickpea Fritters (page 129);
Ratatouille Pasta with Brazil Nut Parmesan
(page 150); Quinoa with Orange-Chilli Kale
and Roasted Butternut Squash (page 146)

Comfort Food

This meal plan is about indulgence – delicious treats to make when you've got a bit more time, such as at the weekend, or for entertaining. These are some of the best recipes to start with when you begin to eat a healthier diet. They're also some of my favourites, and the ones I'd highly recommend for impressing friends and family. And you can round things off nicely with one of my desserts on pages 187–209.

Breakfast: Mini Berry Breakfast Crumble (page 68)
Lunch: Sweet Potato and Leek Soup with Chilli-Roasted Seeds (page 89)
Dinner: Brown Rice Pizza with a Sun-Dried Tomato Sauce (page 156)

Breakfast: Baked Carrot Cake Oatmeal (page 27)
Lunch: Hummus and Black Bean Quesadillas (page 130)
Dinner: Creamy Butternut Squash and Sage Risotto (page 149)

Breakfast: Banana Pancakes with a Blueberry Syrup (page 59)
Lunch: Spiced Carrot, Coriander and Chickpea Fritters (page 129)
Dinner: Lentil Cottage Pie with Sweet Potato Mash (page 154)

Extra Recipes to Pick and Mix
Breakfast: Golden Granola and Coconut Cream Parfait (page 66); Chocolate Porridge (page 44); Quinoa and Chia Bread (page 63) with Raw Chocolate and Hazelnut Spread (page 58); Sassy's Peanut Butter and 'Jelly' Sandwich (page 55)
Lunch: Brown Rice Pasta Salad with Avocado, Rocket and Pesto Vinaigrette (page 106); Ratatouille Pasta with Brazil Nut Parmesan (page 150); Vegan Enchiladas (page 134)
Dinner: Mexican Quinoa, Guacamole and Soured Cream Parfait (page 153); Spicy Squash and Black Bean Burgers (page 144); Sweet Potato and Spinach Dhal with Chickpea Naan Bread (page 141); Chilli Non-Carne with Spicy Baked Potato Wedges and Guacamole (page 131)

FOODS FOR HEALTH

The amazing thing about all the ingredients I use in my recipes is the vast array of benefits they provide. I never thought I'd look at food as something that can help influence the way your skin looks or affect your mindset or your energy levels, but it really has a profound effect on every aspect of our bodies and hence our lives. Knowing this, we can pick foods that are best suited to whatever we're facing on a particular day, to keep ourselves in optimum shape nutritionally, ready to face whatever life throws at us. Below is a list of the foods I've chiefly used in my book – the fruit, vegetables, grains, nuts and seeds – and the specific benefits they each have, often across a whole range of different categories. So next time you're facing a thumping headache, a mid-afternoon energy slump, or a terrible bout of acne – don't despair. Just making yourself a delicious, comforting meal, snack or even drink will do you the world of good! (For information on the amazing benefits of the superfood supplements I use – not included below as they're optional in my recipes – see the Introduction, pages 14, 17–19.)

IMMUNITY: A strong immune system is key for a healthy you. It's so important to make sure you eat food containing a wide range of vitamins and minerals to help to boost your immune system to help it combat infection and illness. These foods are all high in powerful antioxidants, vitamin C in particular, to help keep you fighting fit.

Lemons	Strawberries
Tomatoes	Aubergines
Oranges	Raspberries
Sweet peppers	Quinoa
Pears	Pomegranates
Broccoli	Brazil nuts
Mangos	Pineapples
Red cabbage	Flaxseeds
Apples	Apricots
Sweet potatoes	Pumpkin seeds

ANTI-INFLAMMATORY: Inflammation is the body's natural response to injury or infection, part of a natural healing process, but when it persists or occurs unnecessarily it can cause damage, leading to disease. Everything from headaches, acne and cramp to chronic conditions like heart disease and cancer all thrive off inflammation. Avoiding foods that encourage inflammation (see pages 8–11) and eating an anti-inflammatory diet full of natural ingredients like the ones below will help keep it in check.

Strawberries	Pears
Asparagus	Cashews
Raspberries	Lemons
Avocados	Pecans
Blueberries	Butternut squash
Beetroot	Flaxseeds
Pineapples	Sweet potatoes
Sweet peppers	Ginger
Pomegranates	Celery
Almonds	

ENERGY: Whatever we eat gives us energy, though some foods are better than others at providing a long, sustained stream of energy throughout the day. Unrefined complex carbohydrates and plant-based proteins are ideal, as instead of giving you an instant sugar rush (see pages 10–11), they are digested slowly, keeping blood-sugar levels even.

Pears	Medjool dates
Lentils	Walnuts
Apples	Avocados
Cashews	Pistachios
Blueberries	Brown rice
Almonds	Flaxseeds
Raspberries	Buckwheat
Coconut	Pomegranates
Black beans	Pecans
Bananas	Kidney beans
Peanuts	

RECOVERY: As part of the healing process (see 'Anti-inflammatory' above), inflammation helps muscles recover after exercise, but eating the right foods can keep it in balance, reducing aches and pains and speeding recovery. The foods here will help your muscles heal after a long workout or a strenuous day of activity. They will also help your body recover from physical injury or illness.

Bananas
Coconut
Sweet potatoes
Brazil nuts
Potatoes
Pistachios
Cashews

Kidney beans
Pumpkin seeds
Lentils
Flaxseeds
Quinoa
Black beans
Sunflower seeds

GOOD DIGESTION: Having a healthy digestive system is so important, allowing you to obtain the maximum benefit from the food you eat. When your digestive system isn't quite on track, you'll experience bloating, gas, constipation and a host of other problems in the body. These foods are packed with fibre and hence brilliant for good digestion.

Pears
Fennel
Apples
Celery
Mangos
Courgettes
Strawberries
Aubergines
Raspberries
Asparagus

Apricots
Lentils
Bananas
Oats
Medjool dates
Quinoa
Sweet potatoes
Brown rice
Carrots

HEALTHY HEART: These foods are full of nutrients that will help to maintain a healthy heart by keeping your blood pressure down and your cholesterol levels low.

Oranges
Oats
Fennel
Pecans
Asparagus
Walnuts
Tomatoes
Almonds

Courgettes
Brazil nuts
Chickpeas
Cashews
Lentils
Pine nuts
Quinoa
Pumpkin seeds

STRONG BONES: It's a myth that without dairy products you'll be lacking in calcium; these foods are brimming with calcium and magnesium and other nutrients for strong and healthy bones and joints.

Pineapples
Cucumbers
Broccoli
Chickpeas

Kale
Cashews
Spinach
Almonds

CLEANSING AND DETOXIFYING: Eating foods with an alkalising effect makes for a balanced environment internally (see page 9), helping to rejuvenate cells and allowing your body to function at its best. These foods have a cleansing effect, reducing water retention and removing toxins.

Lemons
Spinach
Limes
Tomatoes
Pineapples
Fennel

Apples
Broccoli
Beetroot
Cucumbers
Kale
Baby leaf lettuce

HEALTHY HAIR AND SKIN: For beautiful hair, clear skin and strong nails, it's not all down to cosmetics. Food plays a huge part in the way we look, and it's all about eating a diet that is rich in healthy fats – omega 3, 6 and 9. These foods will get you glowing from the inside out.

Coconut (oil, butter, milk)
Kale
Cashews
Spinach
Pumpkin seeds
Pecans
Sunflower seeds
Brazil nuts

Avocados
Sesame seeds
Almonds
Butternut squash
Walnuts
Sweet potatoes
Flaxseeds

Fitness and Exercise

Fitness is a huge part of what makes up a healthy lifestyle. While it is vital to nourish your body with the right foods, it is equally important to take enough exercise. Not only does this promote all round well-being, but it also releases endorphins, which are known to give you a buzz of happiness. So not only will regular exercise give you a toned and sleek body, but it will make you feel great too!

Even as a ballerina, I find it difficult to get into my groove with other forms of exercise, so don't be hard on yourself if you haven't yet hit on the best way to work out. Everyone's different, and what suits one person may not suit someone else; the most important thing is to have a go and enjoy it. To supplement my dancing, I love to try different things and give my body new challenges. I've listed a few of my favourite forms of exercise below, as well as a few tips on how to stay active every day.

My Three Favourite Workouts

Ballet

Don't worry – I'm not encouraging you to buy a tutu and a pair of pointe shoes and come to one of my ballet classes (though it would be fun!). Ballet is actually a brilliant form of exercise, no matter how flexible or ballerina-esque you are. It works the muscles in a very different way, and helps add a discipline, strength and control to your fitness regime. There are brilliant adult and beginner classes that take you through the basic movements, which you can then build on. I also really enjoy fitness classes based on the ballet method, such as barre workouts.

Hosted by gyms or training centres, these use the simplest ballet positions to create a hard-core workout.

Pilates

Pilates is something I've always done to supplement my dancing. It's a great way to tone and strengthen your body by focusing on different muscle groups. There are studios everywhere, and often good deals to be had if you sign up for multiple classes. One of the particular benefits of pilates classes is the individual attention you get from the instructor – a great confidence booster when you're starting a new workout regime.

Hot Yoga

Hot yoga is one of my favourite forms of exercise. Consisting of different styles of yoga performed in a sauna-like temperature, this immediately warms the muscles, increases flexibility and helps you take your workout to the next level. I also find it extremely detoxifying, and one of the few things I find really relaxes me after a busy day.

Keeping Active Every Day

Here are five easy things you can do every day to keep your body on the move and those endorphins high!

~ Ditch the lift and take the stairs
~ Get off the tube or bus a few stops early and walk to work
~ Why not cycle, run or power-walk to work instead? It's cheaper too!

~ Attend a lunchtime workout class; loads of gyms offer 30-minute express workouts
~ Use a BOSU ball at your desk; you may feel a bit silly at first, but this is a great way to engage your core all day while you work

Eating to Fuel and Recover after Exercise

As a dancer, I'm constantly thinking of ways I can use food to up my stamina, and help push through a workout. Equally, I'm always trying to give my body the right foods to recover after a workout, too. The key to this is balance. Before and after you exercise, try eating a high-carbohydrate snack with a good balance of protein and healthy fats. An example of this would be a smoothie bowl with banana, oat milk, brown rice protein powder and berries. You could also try my gingerbread or brownie bars (see page 172) or, for a more wholesome snack, gluten-free toast with almond butter. Keep hydrated, and recover with a glass of coconut water. (See also Foods for Health, pages 214–216, and the 'Gym Bunnies' meal plan on pages 210–211.)

Well-being

When we think about health, our thoughts immediately turn to our bodies and we tend to forget the importance of a healthy mind. The way we feel all starts from the top: you want to be sharp and focus clearly, but you also need to wind down and relax. A good balance is key, and something I'm constantly striving for. It's much easier said than done, of course: in this busy world that we live in, our stress levels just seem to get higher and higher, with never enough time to relax. Yet the benefits of taking time out are truly worth it – you feel so much more focused, fresher and able to tackle the day ahead. Stress, in my opinion, is just as bad as junk food; over time it can contribute to serious health problems. Just as I hope to encourage you to make better choices with your diet, it's important to look to your mind too, and take time to unwind properly. My favourite ways to relax are by taking a long bath, doing a hot yoga class (see page 217), taking a 10-minute power nap or having a massage. I try to include one of these every day and schedule it in just as I would a meeting. It can be hard to find the time, but really worthwhile.

Eating to Relax and Rejuvenate

There are certain foods and herbs that can help you relax and feel calm. Lavender, camomile and peppermint are all great herbal remedies for a restless night or a stressful day. Just a warm mug of tea infused with one of these herbs will have a great effect on your body. Another terrific stress-reliever is cacao – the raw form of chocolate (see page 17). Recent studies have shown that it can help to reduce levels of cortisol and catecholamines (hormones associated with stress), especially beneficial for those with high anxiety levels. Try my Superfood Hot Chocolate on page 76.

Natural Beauty

It's so important to think about all aspects of a healthy body. Once I made the transition to eating a much more wholesome diet, I started to get very interested in other ways I could benefit my body, and looked into how what we put on our skin affects our bodies. While we may not eat our face masks, or drink our make-up remover, this doesn't mean they have no effect. In fact, most skin, nail, hair and make-up products are absorbed by the body and into the bloodstream. I now try to buy the cleanest, most natural products on the market, and believe this has totally changed the way my skin feels and how I look. As well as having clearer skin, I feel so much more confident within myself, knowing that the products I buy do me good. I also love experimenting with fun face masks and scrubs made with ingredients from my kitchen. The same foods that are wonderful to eat for a beautiful you are also great applied straight onto your skin or hair.

Below I've shared two of my favourite DIY natural beauty recipes. They're fun, a little messy and totally delicious (not that you should eat them!).

AVOCADO FACE MASK

1 avocado, peeled and stoned
Juice of 1 lemon
1 tablespoon coconut oil, melted
1 teaspoon raw honey, agave or date syrup

Simply pop all the ingredients in a blender and blend until smooth. Alternatively, mash the avocado until smooth and mix in all the other prepared ingredients.

Apply by spreading the mixture all over your face, keeping it on for at least 15–20 minutes. Wash it off with lukewarm water.

COCONUT SUGAR LIP SCRUB

2 tablespoons coconut palm sugar
2 tablespoons coconut oil
1 tablespoon ground cinnamon
1 tablespoon raw honey, agave
or date syrup or well-mashed banana

Mix the ingredients together in a bowl until completely combined. Take about a quarter of a teaspoon of the mixture and gently rub in a circular motion on your lips and any area around your lips that is a little rough or sore. Rinse with warm water, then moisturise with a little lip balm or coconut oil.

You can store this in an airtight container in the fridge.

Eat for a Beautiful You

Beauty starts from the inside out, so focusing on skin-loving Omega-3 fatty acids in your diet is really important for getting that gorgeous glow. For foods that are brilliant for this, see Foods for Health on pages 214–216.

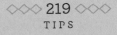

INDEX

Acknowledgements

First and foremost I'd like to thank everyone who's ever made one of my recipes, read my blog or commented on my Instagram posts. Sharing my journey with you has been incredible and I can't thank each and every one of you enough for supporting me and making this book possible.

Thanks to my wonderful editor Laura Higginson for believing in my book, and helping me bring it to life. To everyone at Ebury for all your support and trust, it's been a dream to work with you. My agent Jamie Coleman who helped me realise the book I wanted to write and helped me turn a one-paragraph book proposal into my first book.

Thank you Matt Russell for bringing my recipes to life and making every photograph cover worthy! Ellie Jarvis for making every dish look incredible and always buying the biggest jar of almond butter and extra rooibos tea! Lydia Brun for making every shoot feel like I'd walked into my favourite crockery shop! Smith & Gilmour for turning endless word documents into my first book! Anthropologie Europe and Susie Watson Designs for letting us use your beautiful homeware.

Thank you Jodie Corcoran my amazing assistant at Naturally Sassy. Jose Martin for letting me multi-task and turn my ballet classes into business meetings and strategy sessions! You've been a brilliant mentor in both of my worlds.

Thank you to my best friend Indiana for being with me every step of the way on all my adventures. Thanks for recipe testing the majority of this book, and being the biggest support. Thank you to my greatest friends and sisters Sadie and Layla. Layla, for saying goodbye to those delicious (yet totally unhealthy) brownies we used to devour together. Sadie, for giving me my first opportunity to explore my passion for cookery writing with Hip and Healthy. You both inspire me in every way. To my amazing brother, Tom, who gave me the courage to start my blog, put myself out there and share the Naturally Sassy philosophy. You gave me the confidence to start it all. My brother-in-law Nick for being the most vocal taste tester and never telling me my recipes (even the failures) aren't delicious. My nephew Max for featuring in my cookbook! I can't wait for the day I can make some of these recipes for you too. To Granny Phillipa and Creebo who 10 years ago taught me how to make rocky roads and chicken fingers. What a way I've come! Thank you to Grandma Pat for passing down the cooking and dancing genes! To my Grandfather David, and Lindsay, who have both supported every one of my ventures. I know grandpa would have been so proud of this cookbook. And finally to my amazing parents, Emma and Rupert. Thank you for being with me every step of the way through creating Naturally Sassy and writing this cookbook. Thank you for always taste testing my recipes, and letting me make a royal mess in the kitchen on every ocassion. I couldn't have done it without you.

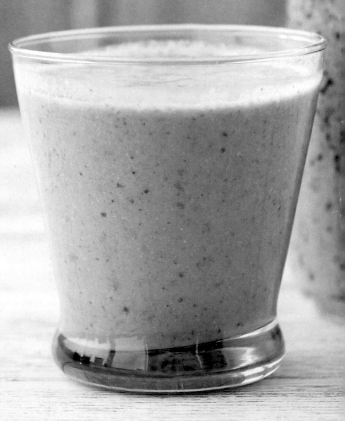